The Complete Healthy Herbal Solution.

300+ Simple Herbal Remedies & Natural Medicines for Everyday Wellness

BY

Love Miner

CONTENT

Introduction

Welcome The Complete Healthy Herbal Solution..

300+ Simple Herbal Remedies & Natural Medicines for Everyday Wellness. This book is more than a mere catalog of plants and their uses; it is a doorway into the world of natural healing, a tradition that stretches across centuries and continents. Herbal medicine represents a deep, rooted connection between humans and the earth, offering powerful, natural solutions to support our health and well-being. In this introduction, we will explore the rich history of herbal medicine, why it remains relevant today, how herbs work synergistically with the body, and the holistic approach to healing that encompasses the whole person—body, mind, and spirit

The History of Herbal Medicine:

From Ancient Cultures to Modern Holistic Practices

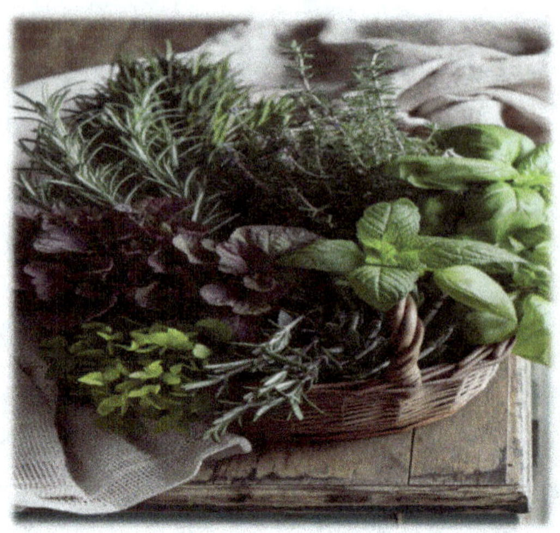

Herbal medicine is one of the oldest healing traditions in the world, deeply woven into the fabric of human culture and survival. Long before modern pharmaceuticals existed, ancient civilizations relied on the natural world to heal and nourish their bodies. Whether you look at ancient Egypt, where herbs like frankincense and myrrh were revered for their medicinal properties, or Traditional Chinese Medicine (TCM), which has relied on an extensive pharmacopeia of herbs for millennia, the use of plants to promote health has been a constant throughout human history.

➢ **Ancient Egypt:** Records show that the Egyptians used herbs such as garlic, juniper, and aloe vera to treat wounds, infections, and digestive issues. The famous Ebers Papyrus, dating back to 1550 BCE, contains more than 700 herbal remedies, revealing the complexity and knowledge of herbal healing in ancient times.

➢ **Ayurveda:** Originating in India over 5,000 years ago, Ayurveda is one of the oldest healing systems still in practice today. It places a heavy emphasis on balance and harmony within the body, using herbs like turmeric, ashwagandha, and neem to restore vitality and treat various conditions.

- ➢ **Traditional Chinese Medicine:** TCM has a long-standing tradition of using herbs to balance the body's energy, or *qi*. Herbs such as ginseng, astragalus, and licorice root have been used for centuries to tonify, balance, and strengthen the body.

- ➢ **Native American Healing:** Indigenous peoples of North America have long relied on the healing power of plants, such as echinacea for immune support and goldenseal for infections. Their herbal knowledge is deeply tied to their respect for nature and the balance of life.

- ➢ **The Middle Ages:** During the Middle Ages in Europe, herbalism thrived, particularly in monasteries where monks cultivated medicinal herb gardens. Sage, rosemary, and lavender were commonly used, not just for healing but also for spiritual and ritual purposes.

Why Herbal Medicine Still Matters:

Natural Remedies in the Face of Modern Healthcare Challenges

In a world dominated by pharmaceutical drugs and quick fixes, why should anyone turn to herbs for healing? The answer lies in the unique strengths of herbal medicine, which complement modern healthcare rather than replace it.

Herbal medicine addresses the **root causes of illness** rather than simply masking symptoms. Many pharmaceutical medications, while effective in treating symptoms, do not always tackle the underlying imbalance in the body that led to the condition in the first place. For example, conventional treatments for anxiety may rely on medications that suppress symptoms, but herbal treatments, like adaptogens such as ashwagandha, can help the body better adapt to stress, bringing long-term relief and balance.

Additionally, many people are seeking **natural and sustainable alternatives** to synthetic drugs, which can come with side effects, long-term health concerns, and even dependency. Herbs offer a more gentle approach to healing, one that works in harmony with the body's natural processes.

> **Chronic Illness:** Many chronic conditions, such as diabetes, heart disease, and autoimmune disorders, can benefit from the supportive role of herbs. For example, herbs like cinnamon can help manage blood sugar levels, while hawthorn has been used to support cardiovascular health.

> **Natural Remedies for Everyday Ailments:** Whether it's a cold, flu, digestive upset, or trouble sleeping, herbal medicine provides a wide range of remedies that can often be found right in your kitchen. Ginger for nausea, chamomile for relaxation, and peppermint for indigestion are just a few examples of how accessible and effective herbal treatments can be.

Building Long-Term Resilience: One of the key strengths of herbal medicine is its role in preventive care. Herbs like astragalus and echinacea can be used to strengthen the immune system, while adaptogens like rhodiola and holy basil help the body adapt to stress, reducing the risk of burnout and chronic illness.

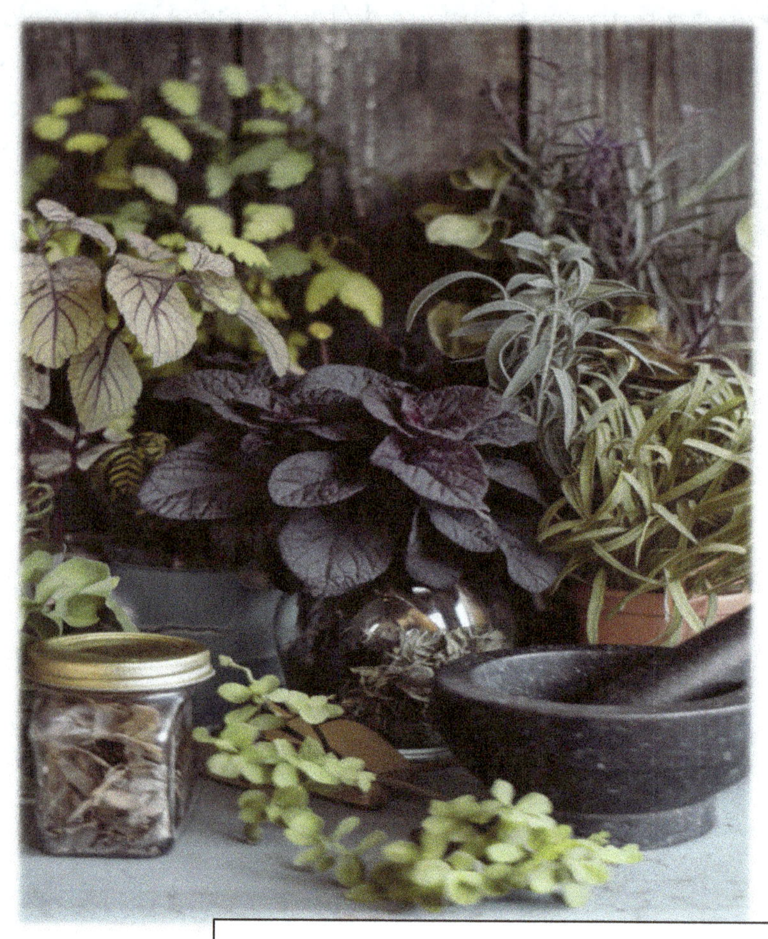

The Complete Healthy Herbal

- effects, herbal anti-inflammatories often nourish the body while reducing inflammation.
- **Antioxidants and Immune Modulators:** Herbs such as green tea and elderberry contain high levels of antioxidants that help fight free radicals, supporting the body in preventing chronic diseases and boosting overall immunity.

Understanding how herbs work within the body is key to using them effectively. Unlike pharmaceutical drugs, which often target a specific symptom or condition, herbs work on a **systemic level**, supporting multiple body systems and promoting balance and healing.

The Importance of Holistic Healing:

Treating the Whole Person—Mind, Body, and Spirit

Herbal medicine isn't just about treating the body. It takes a **holistic approach**, considering the mental, emotional, and spiritual aspects of healing as well. This is why herbalism pairs so well with practices like mindfulness, meditation, and yoga—it seeks to **restore balance** in all areas of life.

- **Mind-Body Connection:** Many herbs influence both physical and mental health. For example, lavender not only has a calming effect on the nervous system but also supports digestive health. Chamomile can help with both insomnia and gastrointestinal discomfort, showing how interconnected our mental and physical states are.

> **Supporting Emotional Health:** Herbs like St. John's Wort and passionflower are traditionally used for their calming and mood-boosting effects, making them ideal for people dealing with anxiety, depression, or stress.

> **Spiritual Health and Connection to Nature:** Herbal medicine encourages us to slow down and reconnect with the natural world. Gathering herbs, making teas, and preparing remedies can become meditative practices that nourish not just the body but the spirit.

> **Self-Empowerment Through Healing:** The act of creating your own herbal remedies can be deeply empowering. It offers a sense of agency over your health and promotes a feeling of independence, fostering a stronger connection to yourself and your body.

Holistic healing doesn't just treat a symptom—it addresses the **root causes** of illness, whether they are physical, emotional, or spiritual. This comprehensive approach ensures that healing is deep and lasting.

Treating the Whole Person—Mind,

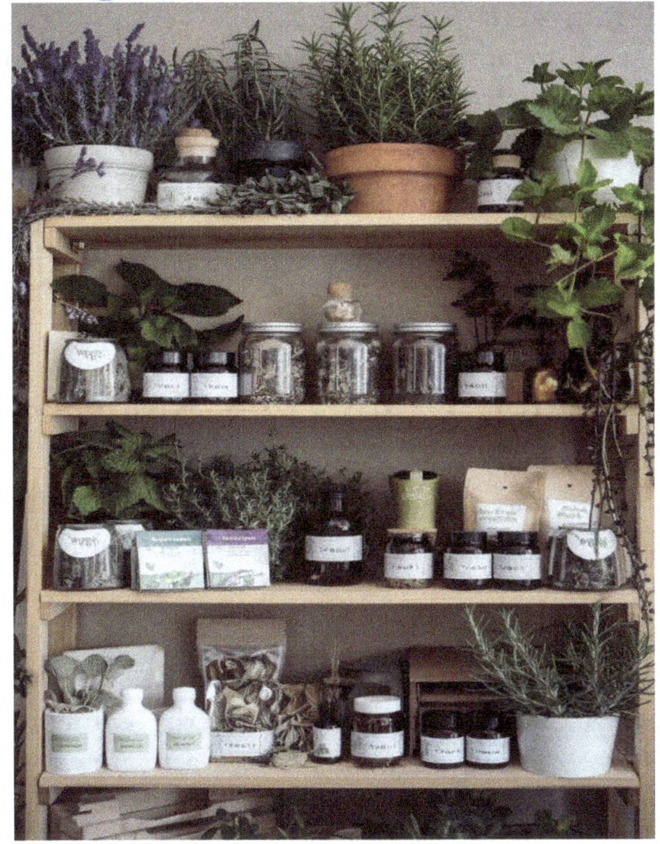

Body, and Spirit

Herbal medicine isn't just about treating the body. It takes a **holistic approach**, considering the mental, emotional, and spiritual aspects of healing as well. This is why herbalism pairs so well with practices like mindfulness, meditation, and yoga—it seeks to **restore balance** in all areas of life.

- **Mind-Body Connection:** Many herbs influence both physical and mental health. For example, lavender not only has a calming effect on the nervous system but also supports digestive health. Chamomile can help with both insomnia and gastrointestinal discomfort, showing how interconnected our mental and physical states are.

- **Supporting Emotional Health:** Herbs like St. John's Wort and passionflower are traditionally used for their calming and mood-boosting effects, making them ideal for people dealing with anxiety, depression, or stress.

- **Spiritual Health and Connection to Nature:** Herbal medicine encourages us to slow down and reconnect with the natural world. Gathering herbs, making teas, and preparing remedies can become meditative practices that nourish not just the body but the spirit.

- **Self-Empowerment Through Healing:** The act of creating your own herbal remedies can be deeply empowering. It offers a sense of agency over your health and promotes a feeling of independence, fostering a stronger connection to yourself and your body.

Holistic healing doesn't just treat a symptom—it addresses the **root causes** of illness, whether they are physical, emotional, or spiritual. This comprehensive approach ensures that healing is deep and lasting.

Safety and Sustainability: Ethical

Harvesting, Proper Dosages, and Avoiding Overuse

While herbal medicine is generally safe when used appropriately, it is essential to approach it with **care and respect**. Not all herbs are safe for everyone, and certain populations—such as pregnant women, children, and those on medications—should exercise caution. One of the core principles of herbal medicine is **using the right herb at the right time** and in the right dose.

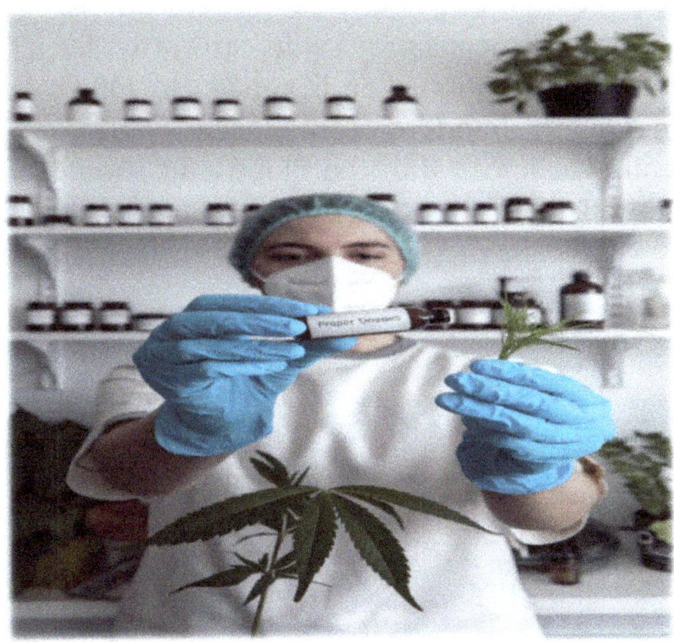

- **Ethical Harvesting**: If you're foraging or wildcrafting herbs, it's crucial to do so in a way that preserves nature. Always leave enough of the plant to continue growing, and avoid over-harvesting endangered species. Sustainability is key in ensuring that herbal medicine can be practiced for generations to come.

- **Proper Dosages**: More is not always better. Overuse of certain herbs can lead to toxicity or adverse effects. For example, while licorice root is excellent for soothing the digestive tract, overuse can lead to high blood pressure. Always follow dosage guidelines, especially when using strong or medicinally potent herbs.

- **Avoiding Interactions**: Some herbs can interact with prescription medications, so it's important to consult a healthcare provider if you're taking medication. For instance, St. John's Wort is known to interfere with certain antidepressants, while garlic can thin the blood and should be used cautiously by those on blood thinners.

- ➢ **Part I: Foundations of Herbal Medicine**: Learn the basics of herbalism, including how to source, grow, and prepare herbs. This section covers everything from teas to tinctures, ensuring you have the skills to start using herbs right away.
- ➢ **Part II: Herbal Remedies for Common Ailments**: This section is packed with natural solutions for everything from digestive issues to immune support, stress relief, and sleep problems. Whether you're dealing with a cold or chronic condition, you'll find practical remedies you can start using immediately.
- ➢ **Part III: Advanced Herbal Practices and Holistic Health**: Once you've mastered the basics, this section will teach you more advanced techniques, like detoxing with herbs, supporting women's health, and enhancing skin and hair naturally. You'll also learn how to build a personalized herbal medicine cabinet tailored to your needs.

Herbal medicine is a journey, one that reconnects us with the healing power of nature. This book will guide you through that journey, offering not just knowledge, but practical, actionable steps to help you integrate herbs into your daily life. Whether you're completely new to herbalism or looking to deepen your practice, this book is designed to support you every step of the way.

Part 1:
Foundations of
Herbal Medicine

Chapter 01
Understanding Herbal Medicine

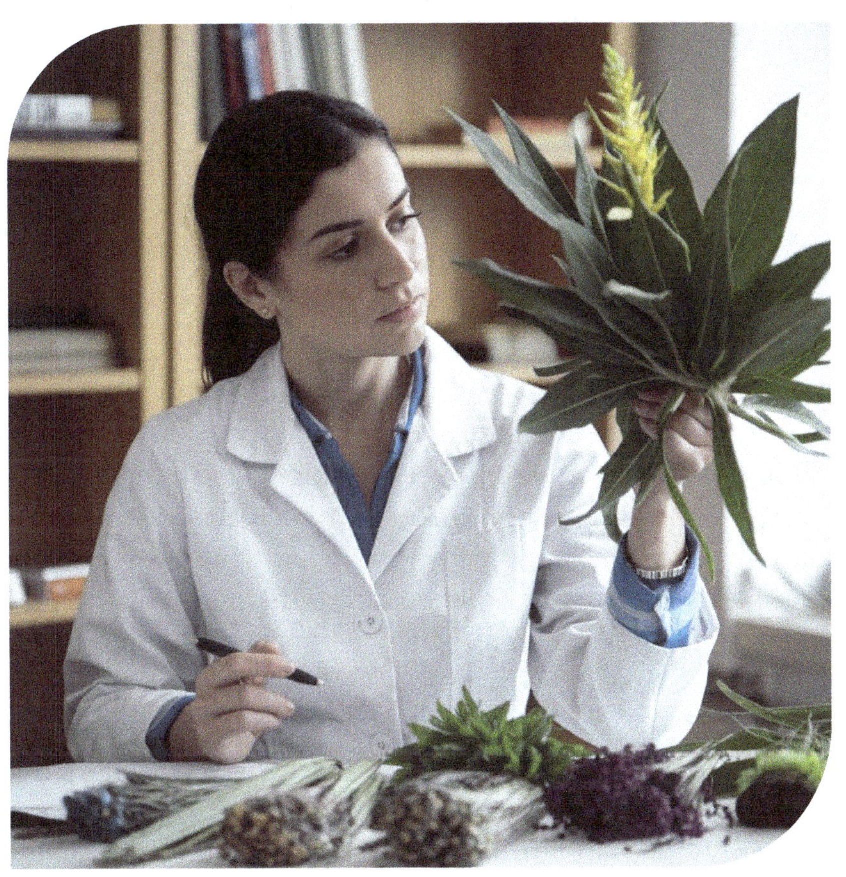

Welcome to the world of herbal medicine! In this chapter, we will explore the fundamental concepts that form the backbone of herbal healing. Herbal medicine is not just a collection of remedies; it's a holistic approach to wellness that respects the body's natural rhythms and encourages healing from within. By the end of this chapter, you'll have a clear understanding of what herbal medicine is, the active compounds in plants, various traditions around the world, and essential considerations for safe and effective herbal use.

What is Herbal Medicine?:

Defining Herbalism and How It Differs from Conventional Medicine

Herbal medicine, also known as phytotherapy, is the use of plant-based substances for therapeutic purposes. Unlike conventional medicine, which often focuses on symptom management through pharmaceutical drugs, herbal medicine emphasizes the use of whole plants or plant extracts to promote healing and maintain health. Here are some key differences between herbal medicine and conventional medicine:

- **Holistic Approach**: Herbalism treats the individual as a whole, considering physical, emotional, and spiritual aspects of health. It focuses on balancing the body's systems rather than merely suppressing symptoms.
- **Natural Remedies**: Herbal medicine relies on the natural properties of plants, using their inherent

compounds to support bodily functions. This is in contrast to conventional medicine, which often employs synthetic drugs that may have side effects.

> **Synergy of Compounds**: Herbs contain a complex mixture of active compounds that work synergistically. This means that the combined effect of these compounds can enhance healing, while synthetic drugs usually target a specific pathway or symptom.

> **Preventive Focus**: Herbal medicine often emphasizes prevention and wellness. Rather than waiting for illness to strike, herbalists advocate for using plants to strengthen the body and boost immunity.

Understanding this fundamental distinction sets the stage for exploring herbal medicine's vast potential as a complementary approach to health and wellness.

Phytochemistry 101:

Understanding the Active Compounds in Plants and Their Effects on the Body

Phytochemistry is the study of the chemical compounds found in plants and their biological effects. These compounds, known as phytochemicals, are responsible

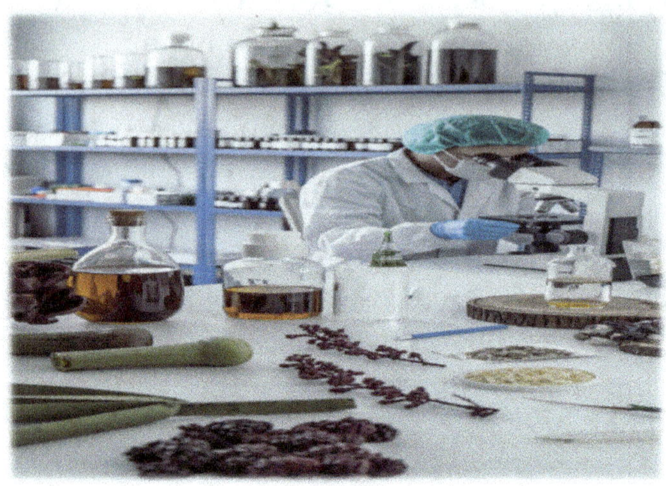

for the medicinal properties of herbs.

Understanding phytochemistry can help you choose the right herbs for specific health concerns and appreciate the complexity of herbal remedies. Here's a closer look at some key types of phytochemicals:

- **Alkaloids**: These nitrogen-containing compounds often have potent effects on the nervous system. For example, morphine from the opium poppy is an alkaloid used for pain relief, while caffeine from coffee stimulates the central nervous system.

- **Flavonoids**: These antioxidants are known for their anti-inflammatory, anti-allergic, and immune-boosting properties. Found in many fruits, vegetables, and herbs (like chamomile), flavonoids contribute to overall health and may reduce the risk of chronic diseases.

- **Tannins**: Present in many plants, tannins can help with digestive issues by reducing inflammation and acting as astringents. Herbs like witch hazel and oak bark are rich in tannins and are often used for their soothing effects on the digestive tract and skin.
- **Saponins**: These compounds can support immune function and may help lower cholesterol levels. They are found in herbs like ginseng and licorice root and have been used in traditional medicine for centuries.
- **Essential Oils**: These volatile compounds provide aroma and flavor to plants and have various therapeutic effects. For example, peppermint oil can help with digestive issues, while lavender oil is known for its calming properties.

By understanding the active compounds in herbs, you can make informed choices about which remedies to incorporate into your health regimen. Additionally, recognizing how these compounds interact with the body's systems can deepen your appreciation for herbal medicine's potential.

Herbal Medicine Around the World:

Exploring Diverse Traditions Like Ayurveda, Traditional Chinese Medicine, and Native American Healing

Herbal medicine is practiced globally, with each culture developing its unique approaches and philosophies. Here's a look at some of the most prominent traditions:

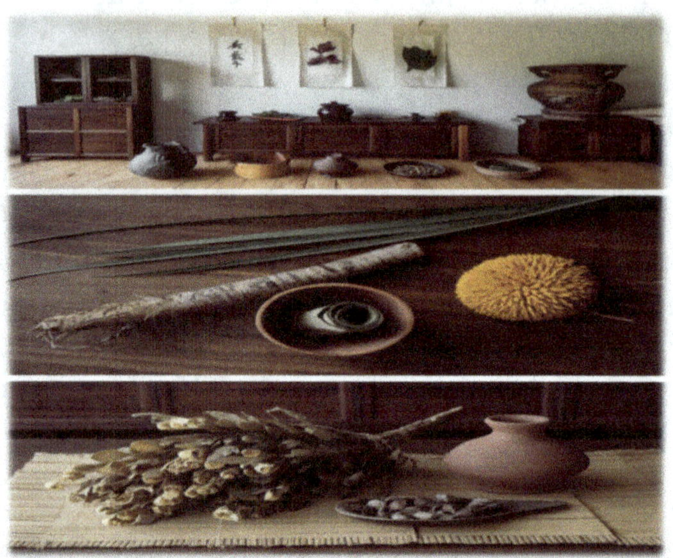

- **Ayurveda**: Originating in India over 5,000 years ago, Ayurveda emphasizes balance among the three doshas: Vata, Pitta, and Kapha. Ayurvedic practitioners use herbs such as turmeric, ashwagandha, and triphala to restore harmony and support overall health. Ayurveda also recognizes the importance of diet and lifestyle in healing.

- **Traditional Chinese Medicine (TCM)**: TCM has a rich history dating back thousands of years. It is based on the concepts of *qi* (energy flow) and the balance of yin and yang. TCM practitioners use a variety of herbs to restore balance within the body. Common herbs include ginseng, ginger, and goji berries, which are used for their tonifying and energizing properties.

- **Native American Healing**: Indigenous cultures across North America have long used herbal medicine as part of their healing practices. Native American healers utilize herbs such as sage, sweetgrass, and echinacea, often in rituals that honor the spiritual connection between humans and nature. Each herb is viewed not only for its physical properties but also for its spiritual significance.
- **Western Herbalism**: This practice blends traditional knowledge with modern research. Western herbalists often focus on using local herbs to treat common ailments. Popular herbs include dandelion, elderberry, and chamomile, which are widely recognized for their therapeutic benefits.

The Body's Natural Healing Ability:

How Herbs Support Your Body's Innate Capacity to Heal

One of the most significant concepts in herbal medicine is the body's natural ability to heal itself. Herbal remedies can support and enhance this intrinsic capacity, facilitating recovery and promoting overall health. Here are some ways that herbs help the body heal:

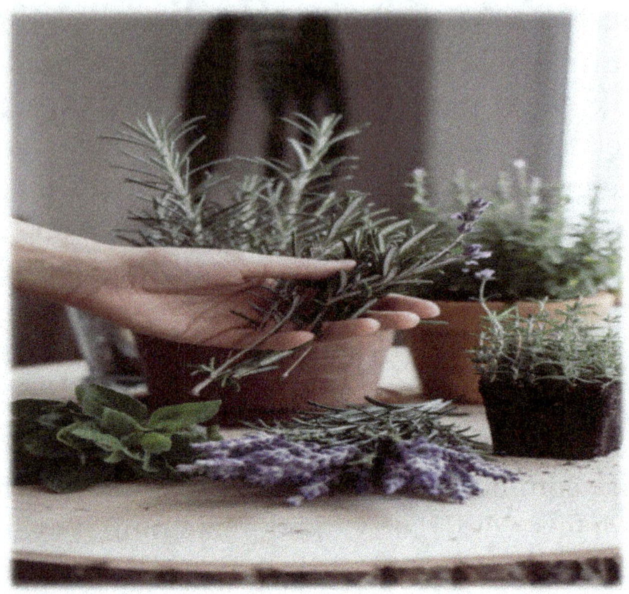

- **Enhancing Immune Function**: Certain herbs, like echinacea and elderberry, are known for their immune-boosting properties. They help prepare the body to fend off infections by stimulating the immune response and enhancing the production of immune cells.

- **Reducing Inflammation**: Chronic inflammation can lead to a wide range of health issues. Herbs like turmeric and ginger contain powerful anti-inflammatory compounds that can help reduce inflammation in the body, supporting recovery from various conditions.

- **Promoting Digestion**: Herbal remedies can aid in digestion by stimulating digestive enzymes and bile production. Herbs such as peppermint and fennel can relieve bloating and discomfort, allowing the digestive system to function more efficiently.

- **Balancing Hormones**: Many herbs support hormonal balance, which is vital for overall health. Herbs like chaste tree (Vitex) can help regulate menstrual cycles, while maca root is known for its adaptogenic properties, supporting energy levels and hormonal health.

- **Supporting Mental Health**: Herbs like St. John's Wort and ashwagandha can help manage stress and anxiety, promoting emotional well-being. By supporting the body's stress response and enhancing mood, these herbs can contribute to overall mental health.

- Understanding the body's natural healing ability emphasizes the importance of a holistic approach to health. Herbs work in tandem with the body's innate mechanisms, providing support and enhancing recovery processes.

Herbal Safety & Allergies:

Recognizing Common Reactions and How to Prevent Harm

While herbal medicine is generally safe for many people, it's crucial to approach it with caution. Allergies, sensitivities, and potential interactions with medications can pose risks. Here are some essential considerations for safe herbal use:

- **Recognizing Allergies**: Just as some individuals may be allergic to certain foods, they can also be allergic to specific herbs. Common allergens include chamomile (related to ragweed), echinacea, and garlic. If you have a history of allergies, it's wise to start with small doses of any new herb and monitor your body's response.

- **Herb-Drug Interactions**: Many herbs can interact with prescription medications, potentially enhancing or inhibiting their effects. For instance, St. John's Wort is known to interfere with antidepressants and birth control pills. Always consult a healthcare professional before combining herbs with medications.

- **Proper Dosage**: Taking herbs in excessive amounts can lead to toxicity or adverse effects. Familiarize yourself with recommended dosages, and avoid using multiple potent herbs

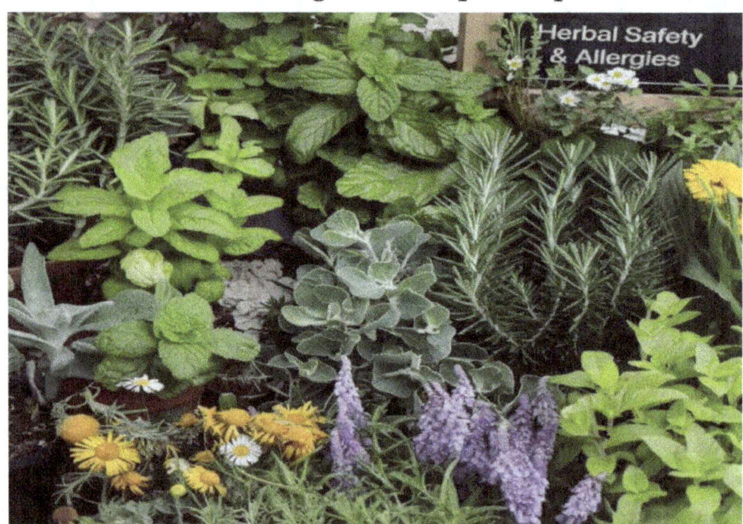

simultaneously without guidance.

- **Pregnancy and Nursing**: Pregnant and nursing women should exercise caution when using herbs, as some can affect fetal development or milk production. Always consult a qualified healthcare practitioner before using herbs during this time.

- **Quality of Herbs**: The quality of herbal

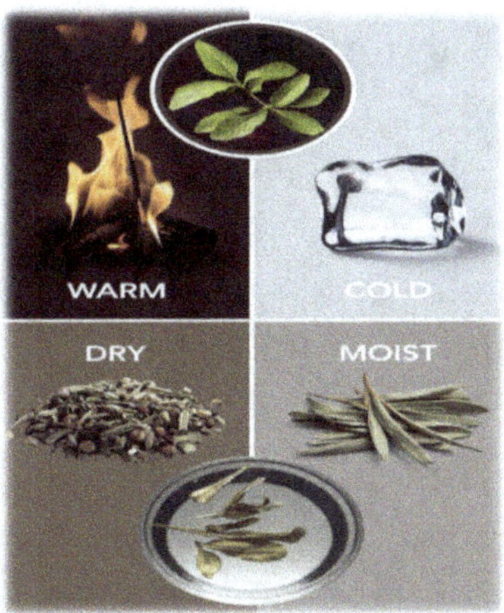

products can vary significantly. Look for reputable sources that provide third-party testing for purity and potency. Freshly dried herbs, tinctures, and teas made from high-quality plants are often the best choices.

Understanding Herbal Energetics:

The Warm, Cold, Dry, and Moist Properties of Herbs

Herbal energetics is a foundational concept in herbal medicine that refers to the qualities and characteristics of herbs and how they interact with the body. These properties—warm, cold, dry, and moist—help herbalists choose appropriate remedies based on individual needs.

- **Warm Herbs**: These herbs tend to increase circulation, stimulate digestion, and promote warmth in the body. Ginger and cinnamon are examples of warm herbs that can be beneficial for cold conditions or for those with sluggish digestion.

- **Cold Herbs**: Cold herbs have a cooling effect on the body, making them ideal for inflammatory conditions or hot flashes. Peppermint and chamomile are considered cold herbs that can soothe overheating and inflammation.

- **Dry Herbs**: Drying properties are important for addressing excess moisture in the body, such as mucus or phlegm. Herbs like thyme and mullein can help reduce congestion and promote clear airways.

- **Moist Herbs**: Moist herbs help combat dryness in the body, such as dry skin or dry cough. Slippery elm and marshmallow root are examples of moist herbs that can provide soothing effects on mucous membranes.

By understanding herbal energetics, you can make informed choices about which herbs to use based on your unique constitution and health concerns.

Conclusion

In this chapter, we've explored the foundational elements of herbal medicine, from its definitions and phytochemical components to the diverse global traditions that practice it. We also discussed the body's innate healing ability and emphasized the importance of safety and herbal energetics. This understanding sets the stage for the practical applications of herbal medicine that you will discover in the following chapters.

Chapter 02
How to Source, Grow, and Harvest Herbs

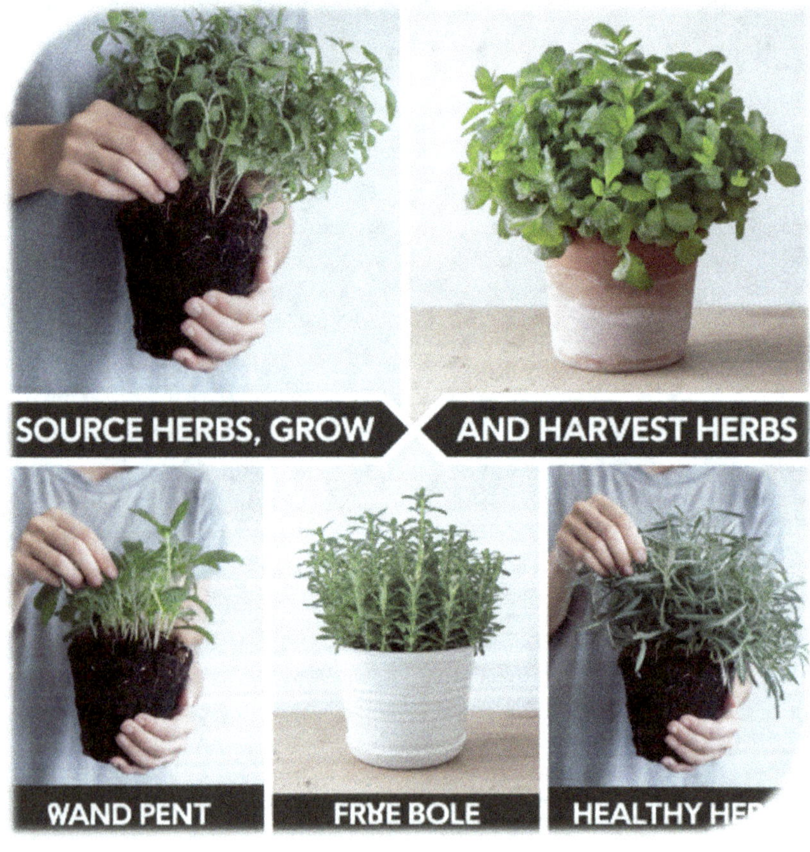

In this chapter, we will dive into the practical aspects of sourcing, growing, and harvesting herbs for your herbal medicine practice. The journey of herbal healing begins with understanding where to find quality herbs, how to cultivate them yourself, and the best practices for harvesting and storing them. Whether you choose to grow your own medicinal garden or forage for wild herbs, this chapter will provide you with actionable steps to ensure you have access to fresh and effective remedies.

Choosing the Right Herbs:

Where to Buy High-Quality Herbs and Avoid Contaminants

Sourcing high-quality herbs is essential for effective herbal medicine. The potency and safety of herbal remedies rely heavily on the quality of the herbs used. Here are some tips for choosing the right herbs:

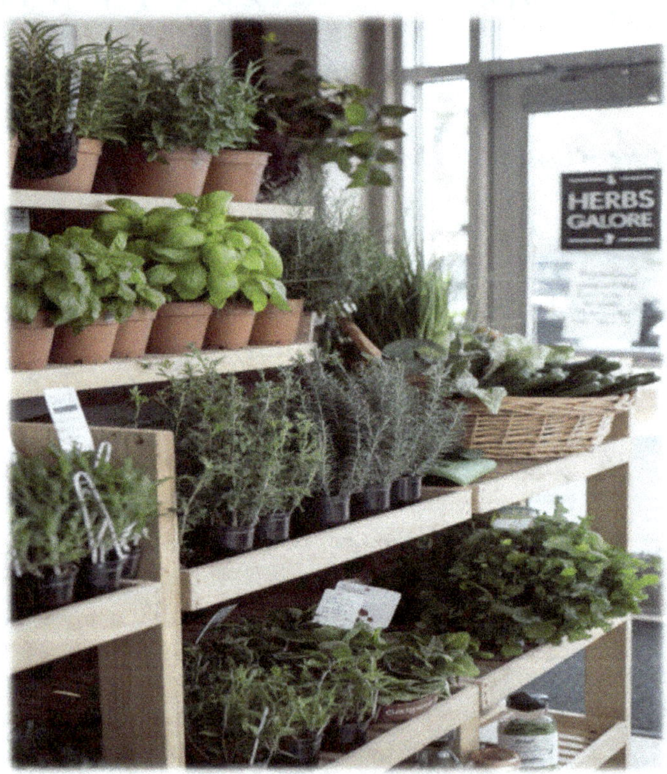

➢ **Research Suppliers**: Look for reputable herb suppliers who have a good track record. Online retailers, local herb shops, and health food stores often have quality herbs. Read reviews and check for certifications to ensure you're purchasing from a trusted source.

➢ **Check for Contaminants**: Herbs can be contaminated with pesticides, heavy metals, or other harmful substances. Look for suppliers who provide third-party testing for their products. Organic certification is also a good indicator of quality, as it typically means fewer chemicals are used in the growing process.

➢ **Buy Whole Herbs Whenever Possible**: Whole herbs tend to be more potent than processed forms like powders or capsules. When you buy whole herbs, you have control over how they are prepared, ensuring maximum freshness and efficacy.

➢ **Observe Packaging**: Quality herbs should be packaged in airtight containers, preferably in dark glass to protect them from light, which can degrade potency. Avoid herbs that are packaged in plastic or are exposed to air.

➢ **Trust Your Senses**: Use your senses to evaluate herbs. Fresh herbs should have a strong aroma, vibrant color, and no signs of mold or spoilage. If purchasing dried herbs, they should not have a dusty or faded appearance.

By taking the time to choose the right herbs, you'll set a solid foundation for your herbal practice.

Growing Your Own Medicinal Herb Garden:

Step-by-Step Instructions for Beginner Gardeners

There's nothing quite like the satisfaction of growing your own medicinal herbs. Not only do you ensure quality and freshness, but tending to your garden also fosters a deeper connection with the plants you use. Here's a step-by-step guide to help you start your own medicinal herb garden:

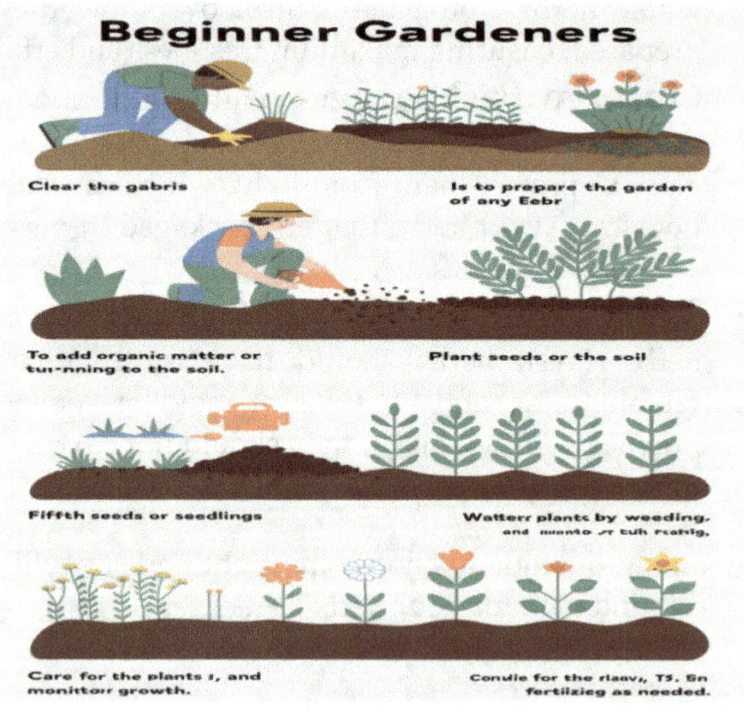

1. Select a Location

> Choose a spot that receives at least six hours of sunlight per day.
> Ensure good drainage and accessibility for watering and harvesting.

2. Decide on Herbs to Grow

> Start with easy-to-grow herbs like basil, mint, rosemary, and chamomile. As you gain confidence, you can explore more specialized herbs.
> Consider your health needs and the herbs that align with those needs.

3. Prepare the Soil

> Use a mixture of garden soil and compost to enrich the soil and improve drainage.
> Test the soil pH if possible; most herbs thrive in slightly acidic to neutral soil (pH 6.0-7.0).

4. Plant the Seeds or Seedlings

> Follow the instructions on the seed packets for planting depth and spacing.
> Water the plants well after planting and keep the soil moist, but not soggy.

5. Care for Your Garden

> Regularly check for pests and diseases. Use organic pest control methods when necessary, such as neem oil or insecticidal soap.

> Water deeply but infrequently to encourage deep root growth.

6. Harvesting Your Herbs

- As your herbs grow, begin harvesting by snipping off leaves or stems. Regular harvesting encourages new growth.
- Avoid taking more than one-third of the plant at a time to ensure continued growth.

7. Enjoy Your Harvest

> Use your fresh herbs in cooking or medicinal preparations, and consider drying some for later use.

Growing your own medicinal herb garden can be a rewarding experience, both for your health and your soul.

The Right Time to Harvest:

How to Know When Your Herbs Are Ready and How to Gather Them

Harvesting herbs at the right time is crucial for maximizing their potency and flavor. Here's how to determine when to harvest your herbs:

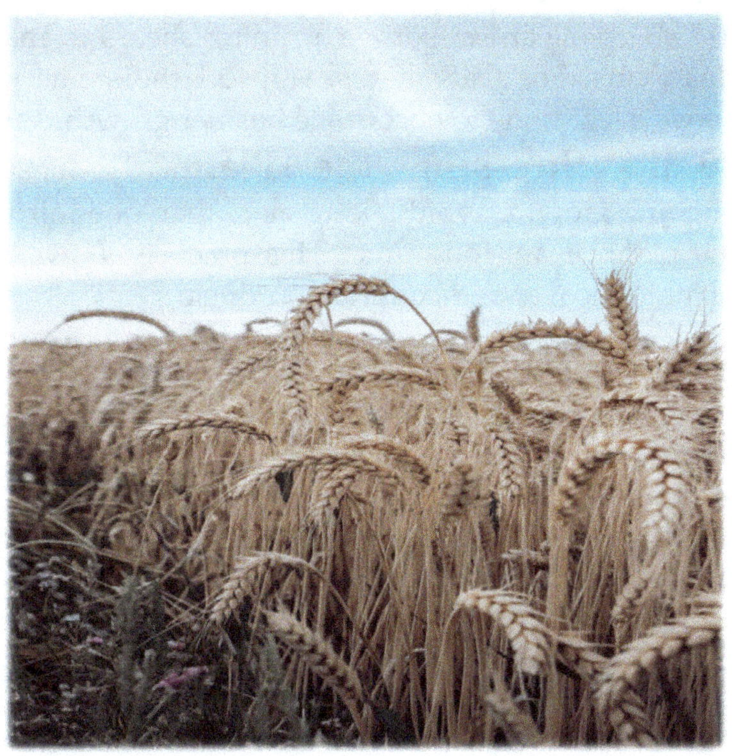

> **Timing Matters**: Most herbs are best harvested in the morning after the dew has dried but before the heat of the day. This timing preserves the essential oils and active compounds.

> **Check for Maturity**: For leafy herbs like basil and parsley, wait until the plant is at least 6-8 inches tall and has developed enough leaves. For flowering herbs, wait until the buds are just starting to open for the best flavor.

> **Look for Color and Aroma**: Healthy herbs will have vibrant colors and strong aromas. If the leaves start to yellow or look wilted, it may be a sign that they are past their prime.

➢ **Use Proper Techniques**: When harvesting, use sharp, clean scissors or pruning shears to make clean cuts. For leafy herbs, snip off the stems just above a leaf node to encourage bushier growth.

➢ **Avoid Stressing the Plant**: To ensure ongoing growth, avoid taking more than one-third of the plant at any one time. This practice allows the plant to recover and continue producing.

By being mindful of when and how to harvest your herbs, you'll be able to enjoy the freshest and most potent remedies.

Proper Drying and Storing Techniques:

Maintaining Potency and Freshness of Your Herbs

Once you've harvested your herbs, proper drying and storage techniques are essential to maintain their

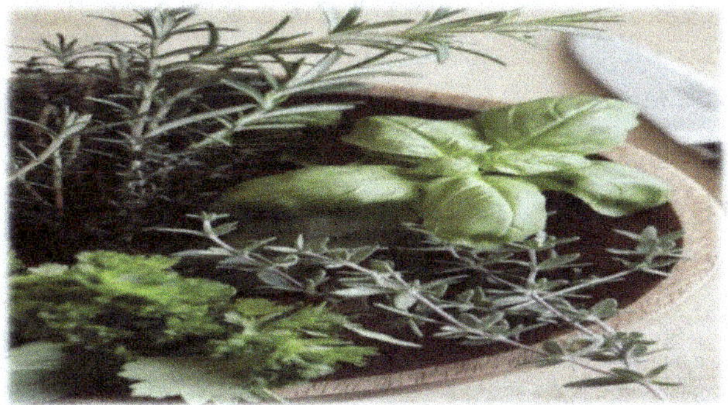

potency and freshness. Here's how to do it effectively:

1. Drying Your Herbs

- **Air Drying**: This is one of the simplest methods. Gather herbs into small bundles, tie them with string, and hang them upside down in a dark, well-ventilated area. Avoid direct sunlight, as it can degrade the herbs' quality.

- **Dehydrator**: For quicker drying, you can use a food dehydrator. Set it to a low temperature (95-115°F) and place the herbs in a single layer on the trays.

- **Oven Drying**: If you don't have a dehydrator, you can use your oven at the lowest setting (around 150°F). Place the herbs on a baking sheet lined with parchment paper and keep the oven door slightly ajar for ventilation. Check frequently to avoid burning.

- **Choose the Right Containers**: Store dried herbs in airtight containers to keep moisture out. Glass jars or metal tins work well. Avoid plastic bags, as they can trap moisture and odors.

- **Label and Date**: Clearly label your containers with the name of the herb and the date it was harvested. This practice helps you keep track of freshness.

- **Store in a Cool, Dark Place**: Keep your stored herbs away from light and heat. A pantry or cupboard is ideal for maintaining their potency.

- **Check for Freshness**: Before using your dried herbs, give them a sniff. If they lack aroma or flavor, they may have lost their potency and should be replaced.

By following these drying and storage techniques, you can ensure your herbs remain effective and flavorful for months to come.

Wildcrafting:

Harvesting in the Wild: Ethical and Safe Practices for Foraging Herbs in Nature

Foraging for wild herbs can be an exhilarating way to connect with nature and expand your herbal medicine repertoire. However, it's essential to approach

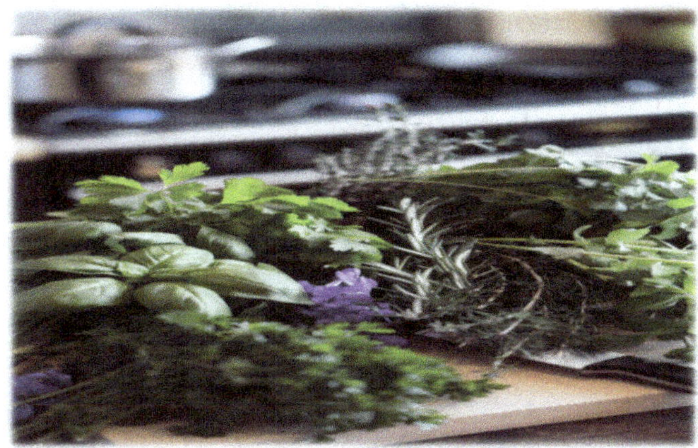

wildcrafting with respect and knowledge. Here are some guidelines for safe and ethical foraging:

- **Know Your Herbs**: Familiarize yourself with the local flora and learn to identify the herbs you wish to forage. Use field guides or apps for plant identification to avoid picking harmful look-alikes.

- **Harvest Responsibly**: Only take what you need and avoid overharvesting. A good rule of thumb is to leave at least 75% of the plant intact to allow it to regenerate.

- **Follow Local Regulations**: Check local laws regarding foraging in public areas. Some places may have restrictions to protect native plants and ecosystems.

- **Be Mindful of Endangered Species**: Avoid harvesting rare or endangered plants. Stick to abundant species that can withstand foraging.

- **Practice Sustainable Harvesting**: When harvesting roots or bulbs, use a digging tool to minimize damage to the plant. For leaves, snip them off rather than pulling them from the base.
- **Leave No Trace**: Respect nature by cleaning up after yourself. Avoid littering and disturbing wildlife habitats.
- Wildcrafting can provide a rewarding experience, allowing you to build a deeper connection with the plants you use. However, it's vital to do so responsibly and sustainably.

Sustainability in Herbal Sourcing:

Supporting Small, Local Herb Farms and Protecting the Environment

Sustainability should be a core principle in your herbal practice. Here are ways to support sustainable practices in herbal sourcing:

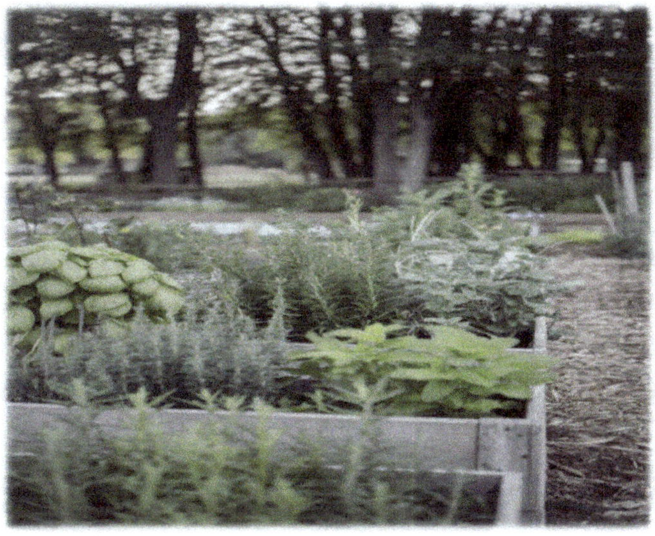

- **Choose Local and Organic**: Whenever possible, buy herbs from local farmers or community-supported agriculture (CSA) programs. Local herbs are often fresher and have a smaller carbon footprint. Organic herbs ensure fewer chemicals are used in their cultivation.

- **Support Small Businesses**: Purchase from small herb farms and local herbalists who prioritize ethical practices over mass production. Supporting these businesses helps maintain traditional herbal knowledge and fosters community resilience.

- **Participate in Community Events**: Attend local herb festivals, workshops, and markets to connect with local herbalists and farmers. These events often promote sustainable practices and provide opportunities to learn more about herbal medicine.

- **Practice Responsible Gardening**: If you grow your own herbs, avoid using synthetic pesticides and fertilizers. Consider permaculture techniques, which focus on creating sustainable and self-sufficient ecosystems.

- **Educate Others**: Share your knowledge about sustainable practices with friends and family. Encourage others to choose responsibly sourced herbs, helping to create a broader impact.

By prioritizing sustainability in your herbal sourcing, you not only enhance your health and wellness but also contribute to the health of the planet.

Chapter 03
Herbal Preparations: Teas, Tinctures, and More

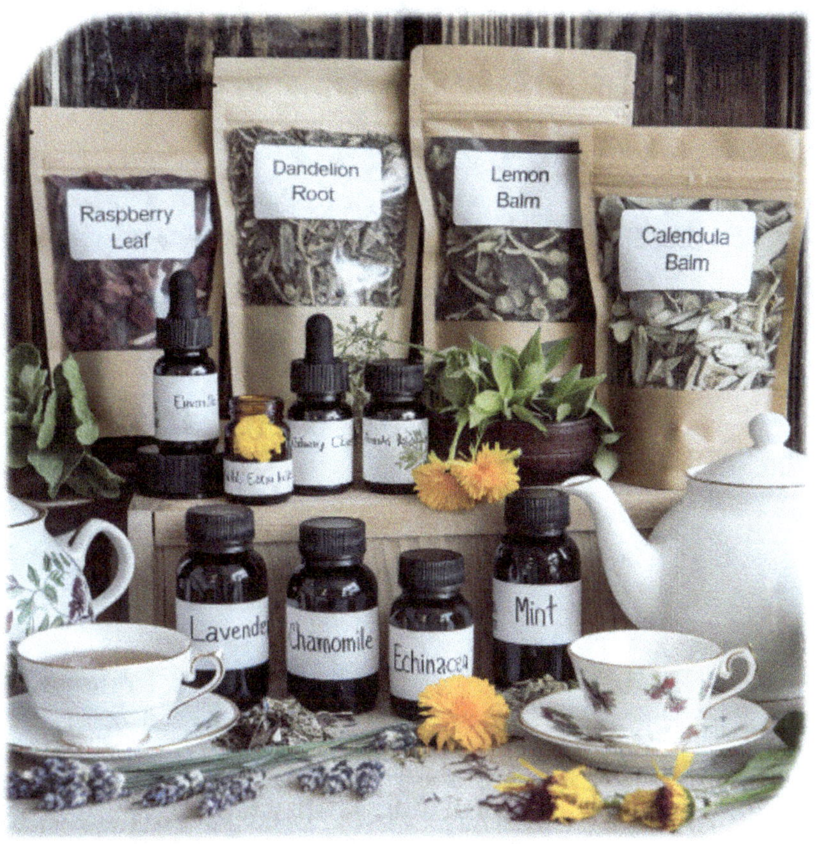

In this chapter, we will explore various methods of preparing herbs for medicinal use. Understanding how to make herbal preparations is essential for harnessing the therapeutic benefits of plants. Each preparation method has its own unique advantages, allowing you to choose the most suitable form based on your needs and preferences.

Herbal Teas and Infusions:

How to Brew Therapeutic Teas for Maximum Potency

Herbal teas are one of the simplest and most enjoyable ways to consume herbs. They can provide therapeutic benefits while also being a soothing ritual. Here's how to brew herbal teas and infusions effectively:

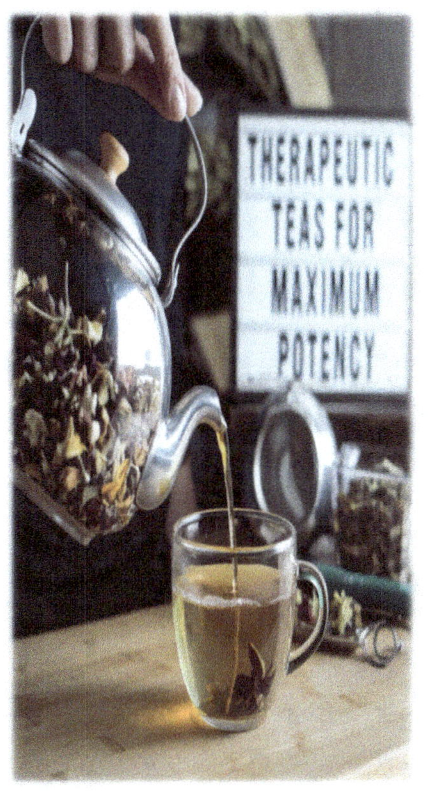
THERAPEUTIC
TEAS FOR
MAXIMUM
POTENCY

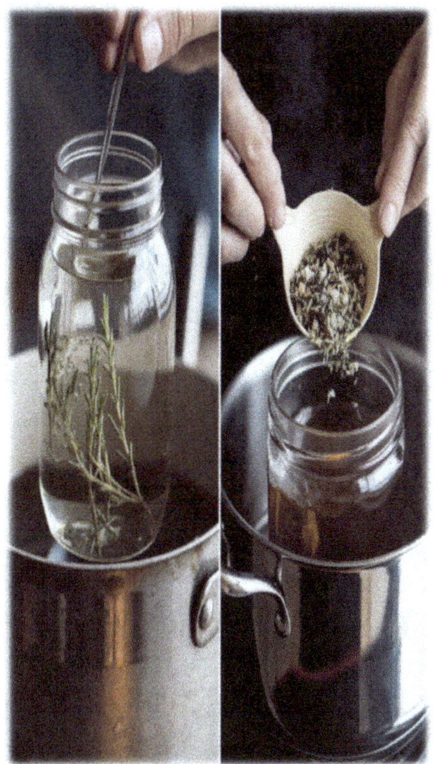

1. Choosing Your Herbs

➢ Select herbs based on their medicinal properties and your health goals. Common options include chamomile for relaxation, peppermint for digestion, and ginger for warming effects.

2. Preparation Methods

Infusion vs. Decoction: An infusion is made by steeping delicate parts of the plant (like leaves and flowers) in hot water, while a decoction involves simmering tougher plant materials (like roots and barks) for a longer period.

Infusion Method:

➢ Use 1-2 teaspoons of dried herbs per cup of water.
➢ Boil water and pour it over the herbs in a teapot or cup.
➢ Cover and steep for 5-15 minutes, depending on the herb.

Decoction Method:

➢ Use 1-2 tablespoons of dried roots or barks per cup of water.
➢ Simmer the herbs in water for 20-30 minutes, then strain.

3. Enhancing Flavor and Benefits

➢ Add honey, lemon, or spices like cinnamon or ginger to enhance the flavor and boost health benefits. For instance, lemon and honey can be soothing for sore throats, while ginger adds warmth and digestive support.

4. Straining Your Tea

➤ Use a fine mesh strainer or tea infuser to strain the herbs before drinking. If you want to retain the nutrients, consider leaving some of the herb particles in the tea, especially for infusions.

5. Storage and Consumption

➤ Consume your herbal tea fresh for maximum potency. If you have leftover tea, store it in the refrigerator for up to 24 hours. Reheat gently before drinking, as overheating can destroy some of the therapeutic properties.

Brewing herbal teas can be a delightful and effective way to incorporate herbal medicine into your daily routine.

Creating Tinctures:

Using Alcohol and Glycerin to Extract Plant Compounds

Tinctures are concentrated herbal extracts made by soaking plant materials in a solvent, typically alcohol or glycerin, to draw out the active compounds. They are easy to use, portable, and have a long shelf life. Here's how to create your own tinctures:

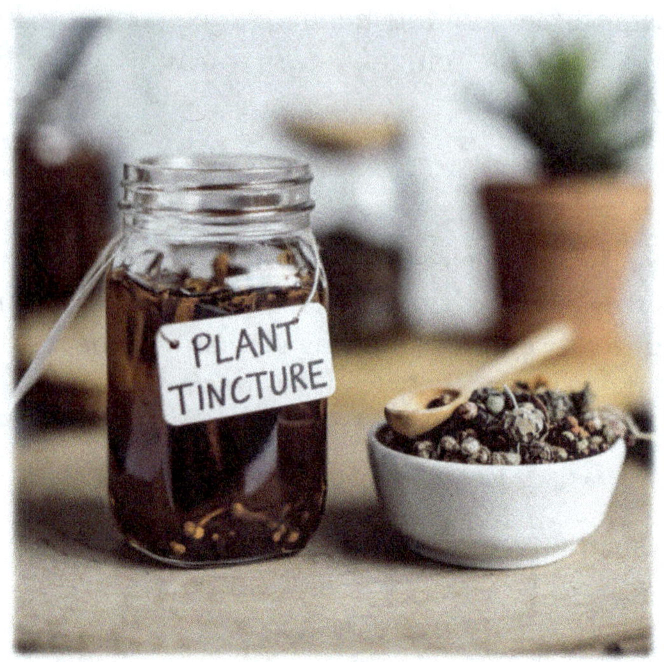

1. Choosing Your Solvent

Alcohol: High-proof alcohol (like vodka) is commonly used because it extracts a wide range of compounds and preserves the tincture effectively. Aim for a vodka with at least 40% alcohol by volume.

Glycerin: A sweeter, non-alcoholic alternative, glycerin can be used to make tinctures for children or those avoiding alcohol. However, it may not extract all compounds as effectively as alcohol.

2. Selecting Your Herbs

➢ Choose herbs based on the health benefits you seek. For example, echinacea is popular for immune support, while valerian root is often used for relaxation.

3. Preparing the Tincture

Ratio: Use a standard ratio of 1 part dried herbs to 5 parts alcohol (1:5) for a standard tincture, or 1 part fresh herbs to 2 parts alcohol (1:2) for fresh herbs.

Procedure:

- ➤ Place the herbs in a clean glass jar and pour the alcohol or glycerin over them until fully submerged.
- ➤ Seal the jar tightly and label it with the date and contents.
- ➤ Store it in a dark, cool place and shake it daily for 2-6 weeks, depending on the herb.

4. Straining and Storing the Tincture

- ➤ After the steeping period, strain the mixture through a fine mesh strainer or cheesecloth, squeezing out as much liquid as possible.
- ➤ Transfer the strained tincture into dark glass dropper bottles for storage. Label with the contents and date.

5. Dosage

- ➤ Tinctures are typically taken in small doses (10-30 drops) diluted in water. Consult with a qualified herbalist or healthcare provider for appropriate dosages based on your needs.

Tinctures are a potent and versatile way to harness the healing properties of herbs and can be easily added to your wellness routine.

Herbal Oils and Salves:

Making Topical Treatments for Skin and Muscles

Herbal oils and salves are excellent for topical applications, providing targeted relief for skin issues, muscle pain, and more. Here's how to make your own herbal oils and salves:

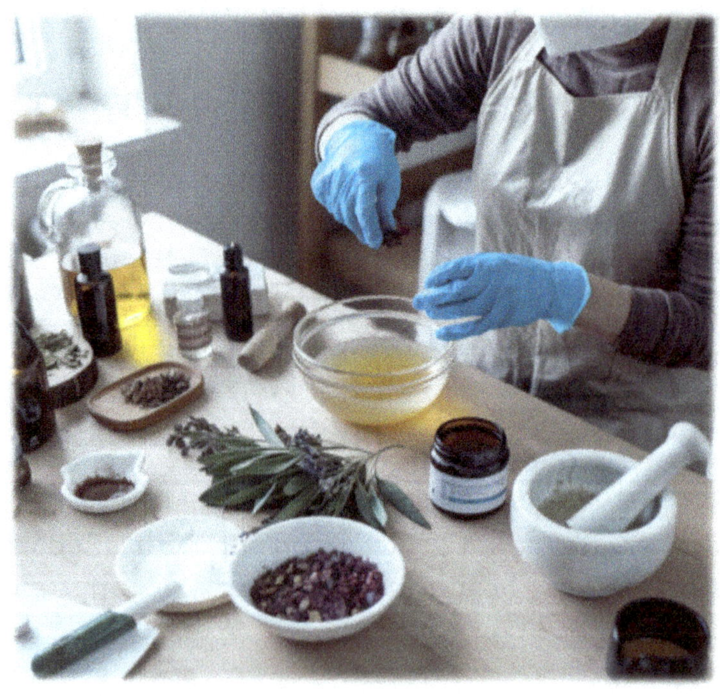

1. Making Herbal Infused Oils

Choose Your Oil: Olive oil, coconut oil, or jojoba oil are great bases for herbal infusions. Each oil has unique properties; for example, coconut oil is excellent for its antimicrobial effects.

Selecting Herbs: Consider herbs like calendula for skin healing, arnica for bruises and muscle pain, or lavender for its calming properties.

Infusion Method:

- Fill a clean glass jar with herbs and cover them with your chosen oil, leaving about an inch of space at the top.
- Seal the jar tightly and place it in a warm, sunny spot for 4-6 weeks. Shake gently every few days to mix.
- After the infusion period, strain the oil through cheesecloth, squeezing out as much liquid as possible.

2. Creating Herbal Salves

Ingredients: To make a salve, you will need your infused oil, beeswax, and optional essential oils for additional benefits.

Salve Recipe:

- Use a double boiler to melt 1 part beeswax with 2 parts infused oil.
- Stir until fully combined, then remove from heat.

- ➢ Add a few drops of essential oil if desired and pour the mixture into small jars.
- ➢ Allow the salve to cool and solidify before sealing.

3. Application

- ➢ Apply herbal oils and salves directly to the affected area. For example, use arnica salve for sore muscles or calendula oil for cuts and scrapes. Remember to perform a patch test before applying new products to sensitive skin.

Herbal oils and salves provide powerful, localized relief and can be a vital part of your herbal first-aid kit.

Herbal Capsules and Powders:

Convenient Methods for Taking Herbs When on-the-Go

For those seeking convenience, herbal capsules and powders offer an easy way to incorporate herbs into your daily routine. These preparations are especially useful for travel or busy lifestyles.

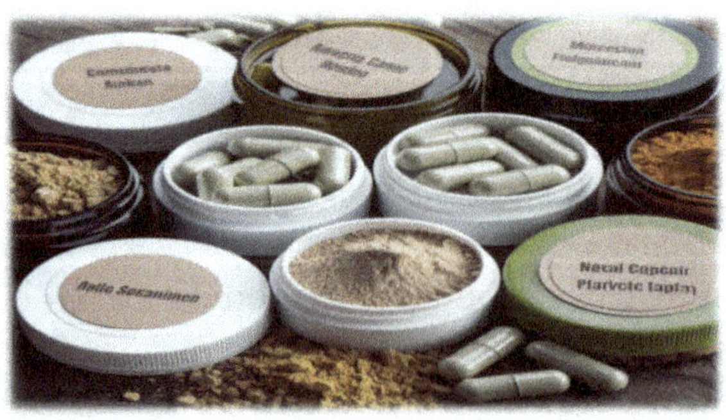

1. Choosing Herbal Powders

➢ Many herbs can be dried and ground into powders. Popular choices include turmeric for its anti-inflammatory properties and spirulina for its nutrient density.

2. Making Your Own Capsules

Gelatin or Veggie Capsules: Purchase empty capsules from health food stores or online. Capsules come in various sizes, allowing you to control dosage.

Filling Capsules:

➢ Use a small funnel or capsule filling machine to fill each capsule with your chosen herb powder.
➢ Store filled capsules in a cool, dry place in an airtight container. Keep them away from light to preserve potency.

3. Using Powdered Herbs

Mix powdered herbs into smoothies, oatmeal, or yogurt for easy consumption. For instance, adding a teaspoon of ashwagandha to your morning smoothie can support stress relief and energy levels.

Always check dosages for each herb, as powdered forms may require smaller amounts compared to teas or tinctures.

4. Benefits of Convenience

➢ Capsules and powders provide a fast and efficient way to incorporate herbal remedies into a busy lifestyle, making it easier to maintain health and wellness on-the-go.

With herbal capsules and powders, you can easily integrate the power of herbs into your daily routine without sacrificing convenience.

Herbal Syrups and Honeys:

Making Palatable Remedies for Cold, Flu, and More

Herbal syrups and honeys are not only delicious but also offer a sweet way to consume herbal remedies, especially for children or those averse to traditional herbal preparations. Here's how to create your own:

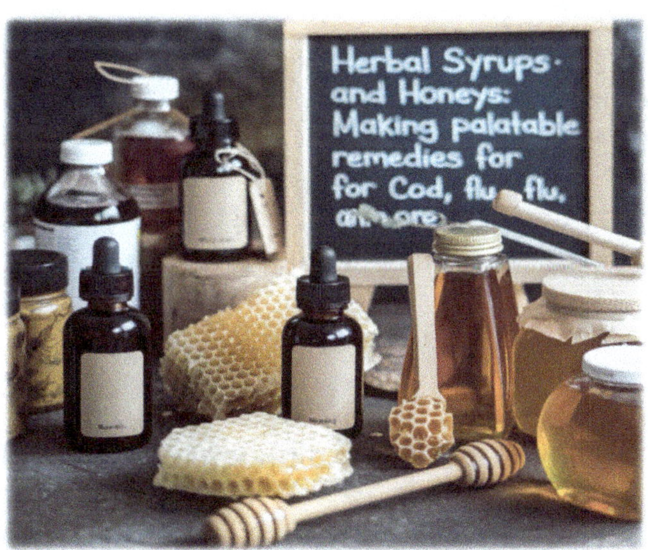

1. Choosing Your Ingredients

➤ Select herbs known for their soothing and medicinal properties. Common choices include elderberry for immune support, ginger for digestion, and thyme for respiratory health.

2. Creating Herbal Syrups

➤ **Basic Syrup Recipe:**
➤ Prepare an herbal infusion by steeping your chosen herbs in boiling water for 20-30 minutes.
➤ Strain the herbs and return the liquid to the pot.
➤ For every cup of liquid, add 1 cup of honey or sugar and simmer gently until dissolved.
➤ Store in a clean glass jar in the refrigerator for up to a month.

3. Making Herbal Honeys

Infused Honey Method:

➤ Fill a clean jar with herbs and cover with raw honey. Allow the mixture to sit in a warm place for several days or up to a few weeks, stirring occasionally.
➤ Strain the herbs before using. This honey can be added to tea or taken by the spoonful.

4. Dosage and Uses

➤ Take herbal syrups or honeys by the teaspoon for cough relief, immune support, or soothing a sore throat.

> These preparations can also be mixed into warm water or herbal tea for a comforting drink.

Herbal syrups and honeys are delightful remedies that not only taste great but also deliver the healing power of herbs, making them a favorite for families.

Dosage and Storage:

How to Measure, Store, and Administer Herbal Preparations Properly

Proper dosing and storage of herbal preparations are crucial for maximizing their benefits and ensuring safety. Here's how to navigate these aspects effectively:

- **Understanding Dosage**

> Always start with lower doses, especially if you are new to herbal remedies. Gradually increase as needed while monitoring your body's response.
> Consult with a healthcare provider or herbalist for personalized dosage recommendations.

- **Measuring Herbal Preparations**

> Use standardized measurements (teaspoons, tablespoons, dropperfuls) for consistent dosing.
> Keep a dosage chart handy for reference, especially for tinctures and concentrated preparations.**Storage Tips**

Teas and Infusions: Store in airtight containers away from light and moisture to preserve freshness. Use within a week for the best potency.

Tinctures: Store in dark glass bottles in a cool, dark place to protect against degradation from light and heat.

Oils and Salves: Keep in a cool, dry place and avoid exposure to heat to maintain integrity. Check for signs of spoilage (rancid smell, discoloration).

Capsules and Powders: Store in airtight containers in a cool, dark place to prevent moisture and light exposure.

Syrups and Honeys: Refrigerate for longer shelf life and label with the date prepared.

● Safe Administration

Consider using a journal to track your herbal usage, noting the effects and any reactions. This will help you tailor your herbal regimen over time.

Always inform your healthcare provider about any herbal preparations you are taking, especially if you are on medications or have underlying health conditions.

By understanding proper dosage and storage techniques, you can enjoy the full benefits of your herbal preparations safely and effectively.

Conclusion

In this chapter, we've delved into the exciting world of herbal preparations, covering everything from brewing therapeutic teas to creating concentrated tinctures and delicious syrups. Each preparation method has its unique advantages, making it easier to incorporate herbal remedies into your daily life.

As you experiment with these various methods, remember to prioritize quality, proper dosing, and storage. Engaging with herbal medicine is not just about the plants; it's about enhancing your health and well-being through thoughtful, mindful practices. Embrace the art of herbal preparations, and enjoy the journey of healing with nature's gifts.

Chapter 04
Herbal Solutions for Digestive Health

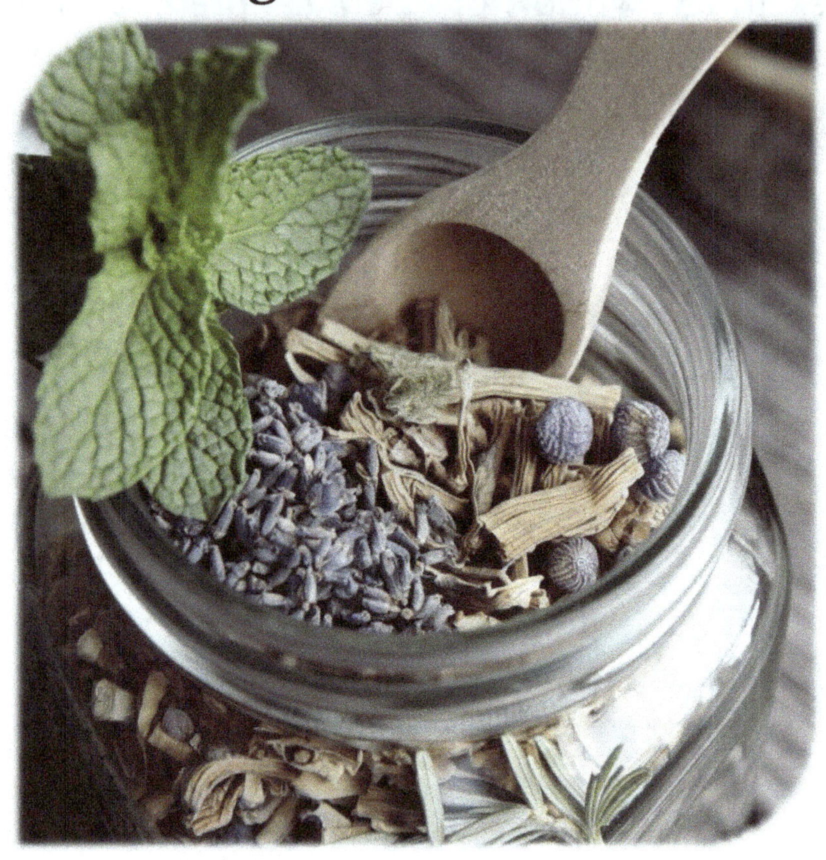

In this chapter, we will explore the remarkable world of herbal solutions designed to promote digestive health. The digestive system plays a vital role in overall well-being, impacting not just our physical health but also our emotional and mental states. Many people experience digestive issues, from occasional discomfort to chronic conditions. Fortunately, nature offers a wealth of herbs that can help soothe, stimulate, and support our digestive systems. Let's delve into various herbs and their benefits for digestive health.

Soothing the Gut with Demulcent Herbs

Demulcent herbs are known for their soothing properties, making them excellent allies for individuals dealing with irritation in the digestive tract. These herbs form a protective layer over the mucous membranes, providing relief from discomfort.

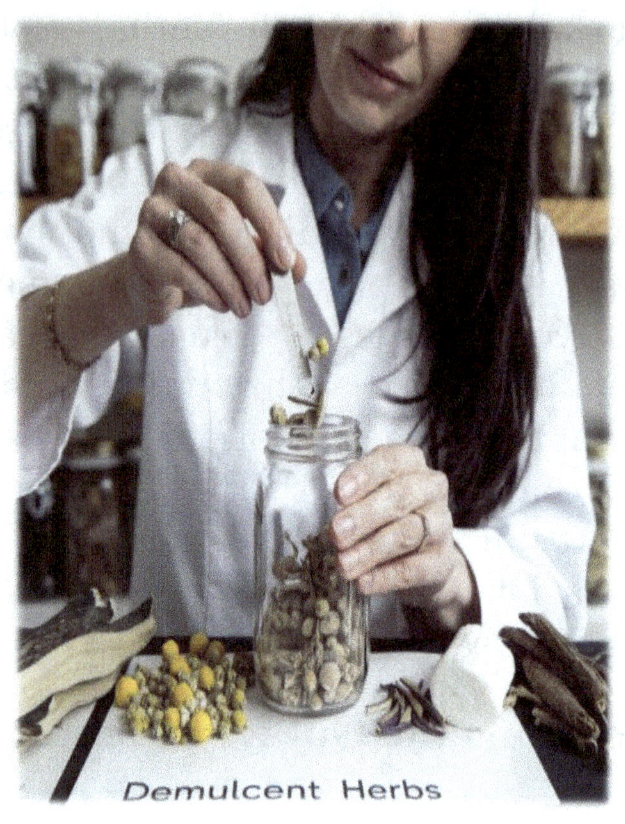

Demulcent Herbs

1. Marshmallow Root

Properties: Marshmallow root contains mucilage, a gel-like substance that coats the digestive tract, soothing irritation and inflammation.

How to Use:

- ➢ **Tea**: Prepare a tea by steeping 1-2 teaspoons of dried marshmallow root in hot water for 15-20 minutes. Drink up to three times a day.
- ➢ **Tincture**: Use 1-2 dropperfuls of marshmallow tincture as needed.

Benefits: Particularly beneficial for conditions like gastritis or esophagitis, marshmallow root helps reduce inflammation and promote healing.

2. Licorice Root

Properties: Licorice root has anti-inflammatory and soothing effects, making it helpful for gastrointestinal issues.

How to Use:

- ➢ **Tea**: Brew a tea using 1-2 teaspoons of dried licorice root. Steep for 10-15 minutes and consume 1-2 times daily.
- ➢ **Tincture**: Incorporate 1-2 dropperfuls of licorice tincture into your routine.

Benefits: Licorice is especially effective in soothing stomach ulcers and reducing inflammation in the digestive tract.

3. Slippery Elm

Properties: Like marshmallow root, slippery elm is rich in mucilage, which coats and protects the digestive lining.

How to Use:

- ➤ **Tea**: Mix 1 tablespoon of slippery elm powder in a cup of warm water. Stir well and drink once or twice daily.
- ➤ **Powder**: You can also take slippery elm in powder form mixed with honey.

Benefits: This herb is useful for soothing sore throats, easing digestive discomfort, and managing conditions like Crohn's disease.

Incorporating these demulcent herbs into your daily routine can significantly benefit your gut health, providing relief from irritation and discomfort.

Bitters for Better Digestion

Bitter herbs stimulate digestion by promoting the secretion of digestive enzymes and bile, which can enhance nutrient absorption and overall digestive function.

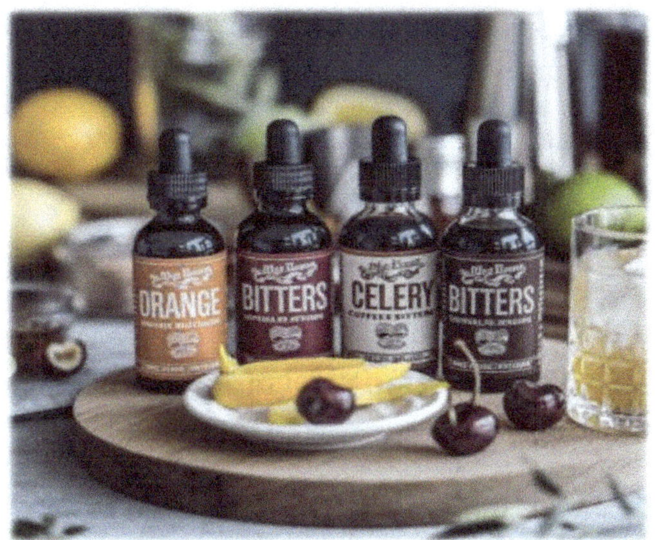

1. Gentian

Properties: Gentian root is one of the most potent bitter herbs and is traditionally used to support digestive health.

How to Use:

> **Tincture**: Take 1-2 dropperfuls of gentian tincture before meals to stimulate digestion.

> **Tea**: Brew a tea using 1 teaspoon of dried gentian root steeped in hot water for 10 minutes.

Benefits: Gentian can enhance appetite, relieve indigestion, and improve overall digestive efficiency.

2. Dandelion

Properties: Dandelion leaves and roots are excellent bitters that promote bile production and liver health.

How to Use:

> **Tea**: Steep 1-2 teaspoons of dried dandelion root or leaves in hot water for 10-15 minutes. Drink before meals.
> **Salad**: Add fresh dandelion greens to salads for a nutritional boost.

Benefits: Dandelion helps with digestion, reduces bloating, and supports liver function, making it a versatile herb for digestive health.

3. Artichoke Leaf

Properties: Artichoke leaf extract is another excellent bitter herb known for its digestive-supportive properties.

How to Use:

> **Capsules**: Take artichoke leaf capsules according to the package directions.

➢ **Tincture**: Use 1-2 dropperfuls of tincture before meals.

Benefits: Artichoke can help reduce symptoms of indigestion and promote bile production, enhancing fat digestion.

Using bitters before meals can stimulate your digestive system and improve the overall process of digestion.

Herbs for Gas and Bloating

Gas and bloating can be uncomfortable and distressing. Fortunately, several herbs can help alleviate these issues by promoting digestive ease and reducing discomfort.

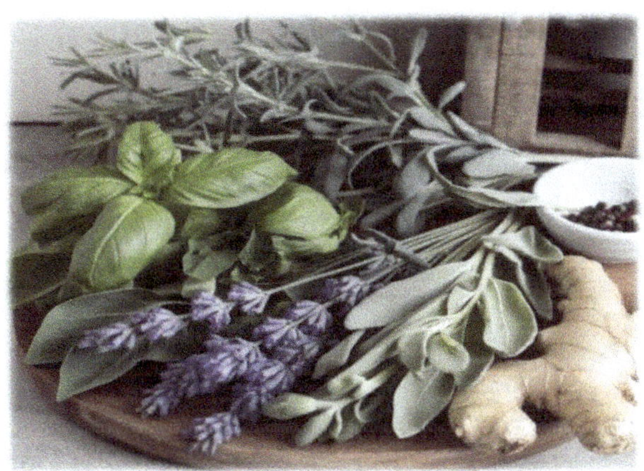

1. Fennel Seeds

Properties: Fennel seeds are carminative, meaning they help relieve gas and bloating.

How to Use:

> ➤ **Tea**: Steep 1 teaspoon of crushed fennel seeds in hot water for 10-15 minutes. Drink after meals to aid digestion.
> ➤ **Chew**: Chew on a teaspoon of fennel seeds after meals to help with digestion and freshen breath.

Benefits: Fennel is effective in reducing bloating and gas while also promoting overall digestive health.

2. Ginger

Properties: Ginger is known for its ability to soothe the stomach and promote healthy digestion.

How to Use:

> ➤ **Tea**: Brew ginger tea by steeping fresh ginger slices in hot water for 10 minutes. Drink before or after meals.
> ➤ **Powder**: Add ginger powder to smoothies or meals for an added digestive boost.

Benefits: Ginger can help alleviate nausea, gas, and bloating, making it a great option for digestive support.

3. Peppermint

Properties: Peppermint is another carminative herb that helps relax the digestive tract muscles, reducing gas and bloating.

How to Use:

- **Tea**: Steep fresh or dried peppermint leaves in hot water for 5-10 minutes. Drink as needed.
- **Capsules**: Consider taking peppermint oil capsules for convenience.

Benefits: Peppermint can provide quick relief from gas and bloating, and it may also help with symptoms of irritable bowel syndrome (IBS).

Incorporating these herbs into your routine can help you manage and alleviate gas and bloating effectively.

Herbal Support for IBS and Chronic Digestive Issues

Irritable bowel syndrome (IBS) and chronic digestive issues can be challenging to manage. However, specific herbs can provide supportive care and promote a more balanced digestive system.

1. Peppermint

Properties: As previously mentioned, peppermint relaxes digestive muscles, making it particularly effective for IBS symptoms.

How to Use:

> **Tea**: Drink peppermint tea regularly to alleviate IBS symptoms.
> **Enteric-coated capsules**: These can deliver the benefits of peppermint oil directly to the intestines.

Benefits: Peppermint can reduce abdominal pain, gas, and bloating associated with IBS.

2. Chamomile

Properties: Chamomile is gentle yet effective, known for its calming and anti-inflammatory properties.

How to Use:

> **Tea**: Brew chamomile tea by steeping dried flowers in hot water for 5-10 minutes. Drink before bed to promote relaxation.
> **Tincture**: Take chamomile tincture for added digestive support.
> **Benefits**: Chamomile can help ease digestive discomfort, reduce inflammation, and promote relaxation.

3. Slippery Elm

Properties: As a demulcent, slippery elm can soothe and protect the digestive lining.

How to Use:

- ➤ **Tea**: Prepare slippery elm tea by mixing 1 tablespoon of powder in warm water. Drink 1-2 times daily.
- ➤ **Powder**: You can also take slippery elm powder directly or mix it with honey.

Benefits: Slippery elm can help reduce symptoms of IBS by soothing inflammation in the digestive tract.

4. Ginger

Properties: Ginger can help ease nausea and digestive discomfort, making it suitable for managing IBS symptoms.

How to Use:

- ➤ **Tea**: Drink ginger tea regularly for digestive support.
- ➤ **Supplement**: Consider taking ginger capsules as directed.

Benefits: Ginger helps with digestion and can alleviate nausea and discomfort associated with IBS.

By incorporating these herbs into your diet, you can find natural support for IBS and other chronic digestive issues, promoting balance and comfort in your digestive system.

72

Herbs for Acid Reflux

Acid reflux can be a painful and disruptive condition. Fortunately, several herbs can provide relief by soothing the digestive tract and balancing stomach acid levels.

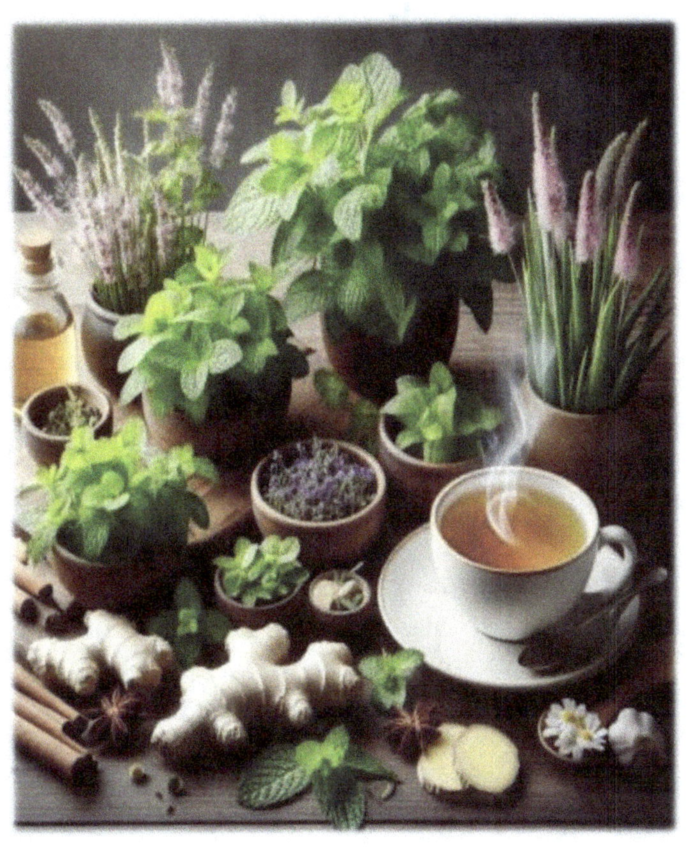

1. Chamomile

Properties: Chamomile is well-known for its calming effects and can help reduce inflammation in the digestive tract.

How to Use:

- ➢ **Tea**: Brew chamomile tea and drink after meals to soothe the stomach.
- ➢ **Tincture**: Consider taking a chamomile tincture for additional benefits.

Benefits: Chamomile can help relieve symptoms of acid reflux and promote overall digestive comfort.

2. Licorice Root

Properties: Licorice root contains compounds that can help soothe and protect the stomach lining.

How to Use:

- ➢ **Tea**: Brew a tea with dried licorice root, consuming it after meals.
- ➢ **Deglycyrrhizinated Licorice (DGL)**: For those concerned about blood pressure, consider DGL supplements.

Benefits: Licorice root can help reduce irritation and promote healing in the stomach lining, alleviating acid reflux symptoms.

3. Slippery Elm

Properties: The mucilage in slippery elm coats the stomach lining, providing relief from irritation.

How to Use:

> **Tea**: Mix slippery elm powder in warm water and drink before meals.
> **Powder**: Take slippery elm powder mixed with honey for additional flavor

Benefits: Slippery elm can soothe the esophagus and reduce the discomfort associated with acid reflux.

4. Marshmallow Root

Properties: Similar to slippery elm, marshmallow root provides a protective layer over the digestive lining.

How to Use:

> **Tea**: Brew a tea with marshmallow root and drink after meals.
> **Tincture**: Use marshmallow tincture for quick relief.

Benefits: Marshmallow root can help calm the digestive tract and reduce irritation from acid reflux.

Incorporating these soothing herbs into your daily routine can provide effective relief from acid reflux and promote overall digestive health.

Supporting Liver Function with Herbs

A healthy liver is essential for optimal digestion and detoxification. Certain herbs can support liver function, enhancing its ability to process and eliminate toxins.

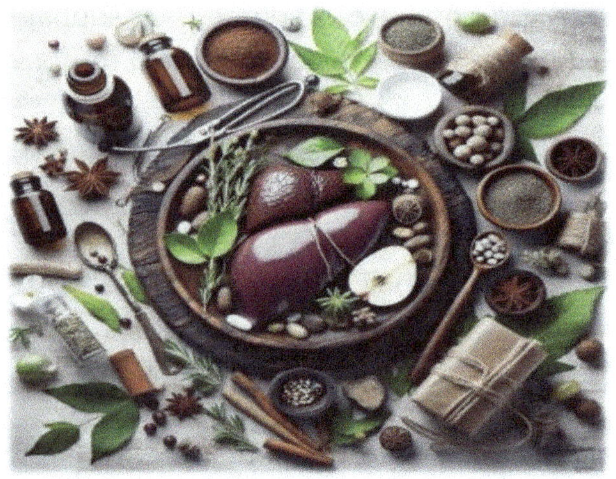

1. Milk Thistle

Properties: Milk thistle is known for its liver-protective properties, primarily due to the active compound silymarin.

How to Use:

> **Capsules**: Take milk thistle capsules according to the package directions.
> **Tea**: Brew a tea using dried milk thistle seeds, steeping for 10-15 minutes.

Benefits: Milk thistle helps regenerate liver cells and protect against damage, making it a powerful ally for liver health.

2. Burdock Root

Properties: Burdock root is a blood purifier that supports liver and kidney function.

How to Use:

> **Tea**: Steep dried burdock root in hot water for 10-15 minutes and drink 1-2 times daily.
> **Powder**: Incorporate burdock root powder into smoothies or soups.

Benefits: Burdock root helps detoxify the body and supports healthy digestion and liver function.

3. Dandelion Root

Properties: Dandelion root is another excellent herb for liver health and digestion.

How to Use:

➢ **Tea**: Brew a tea with dried dandelion root and drink before meals.

➢ **Tincture**: Use a dandelion tincture for additional benefits.

Benefits: Dandelion supports bile production, promoting digestion and detoxification.

Incorporating these herbs into your diet can enhance liver function, improve digestion, and promote overall health.

Conclusion

Herbal solutions for digestive health offer a natural and effective approach to managing a range of digestive issues. From soothing the gut with demulcent herbs to stimulating digestion with bitters, each herb plays a unique role in supporting digestive function. By understanding how to use these herbs and incorporating them into your daily routine, you can foster better digestion and overall well-being.

As you explore these herbal remedies, remember to listen to your body and consult with a healthcare provider if you have any concerns. Embrace the healing power of herbs and nurture your digestive health naturally.

Chapter 05
Herbs for Immune System Support

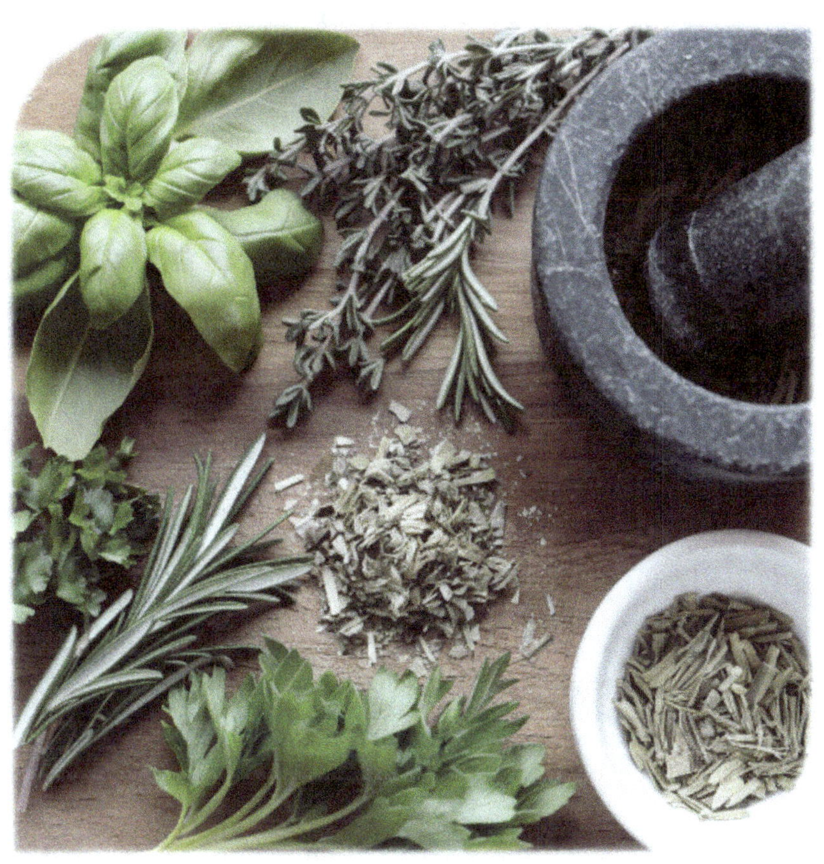

The immune system is our body's frontline defense against infections and diseases. A strong immune response is crucial for maintaining health and preventing illness. Fortunately, herbal medicine offers a variety of potent herbs that can help boost and support immune function. In this chapter, we will explore several key herbs that enhance immune health, combat infections, and promote overall well-being.

TheEchinacea and Elderberry:

How to Boost Your Immune Response Naturally

Echinacea and elderberry are two of the most popular herbs for enhancing immune function, especially during cold and flu season. They have been used for centuries in traditional medicine and are known for their impressive immune-boosting properties.

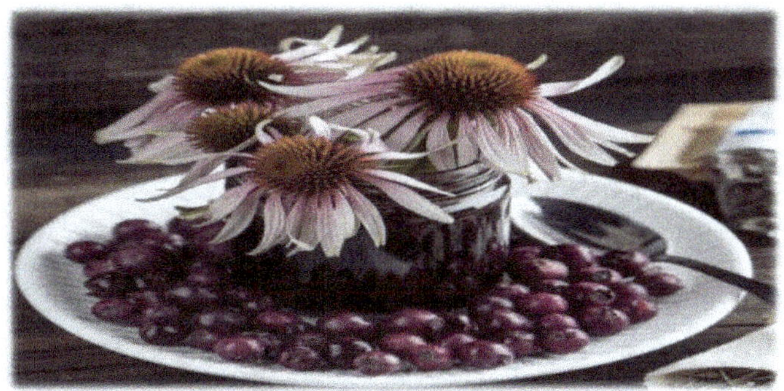

1. Echinacea

Properties: Echinacea is well-known for its ability to stimulate the immune system and reduce the severity and duration of colds.

How to Use:

- ➤ **Tea**: Brew echinacea tea using 1-2 teaspoons of dried root or flowers steeped in hot water for 10-15 minutes. Drink 2-3 times daily during cold and flu season.
- ➤ **Tincture**: Take 1-2 dropperfuls of echinacea tincture at the onset of symptoms.

Benefits: Echinacea enhances the production of white blood cells and activates immune responses, making it effective against respiratory infections.

2. Elderberry

Properties: Elderberry is rich in antioxidants and vitamins, particularly vitamin C, which is crucial for immune health.

How to Use:

> **Syrup**: Elderberry syrup is a popular preparation; take 1-2 tablespoons daily for prevention or 1 tablespoon every few hours when sick.
> **Tea**: Steep dried elderberries in hot water to make a soothing tea.

Benefits: Elderberry has been shown to reduce the duration and severity of influenza, making it a powerful ally in immune support.

Combining echinacea and elderberry can provide a robust defense against colds and flu, helping to keep your immune system strong.

Antiviral Herbs for Colds and Flu

When it comes to fighting viruses, certain herbs have demonstrated antiviral properties that can help combat colds and flu effectively.

1. Oregano

Properties: Oregano contains carvacrol and thymol, which have strong antiviral and antibacterial properties.

How to Use:

> **Oil**: Use oregano essential oil diluted in a carrier oil or take as a supplement, following the recommended dosage.
> **Tea**: Brew oregano tea using fresh or dried leaves.

Benefits: Oregano can help inhibit the growth of viruses, making it a valuable herb for respiratory infections.

2. Thyme

Properties: Thyme is a powerful antiseptic and contains thymol, which has antiviral properties.

How to Use:

- **Tea**: Steep fresh or dried thyme in hot water for 10-15 minutes. Drink 2-3 times daily during cold and flu season.
- **Oil**: Thyme essential oil can be used in a diffuser or diluted for topical application.

Benefits: Thyme helps to relieve cough and congestion while providing antiviral support against respiratory infections.

3. Garlic

Properties: Garlic has long been hailed for its immune-boosting and antimicrobial properties.

How to Use:

- **Raw**: Consume raw garlic by crushing it and adding it to food or drinks.

➢ **Supplement**: Take garlic capsules or extract for a concentrated dose.

Benefits: Garlic enhances the immune response and has antiviral effects, making it an effective natural remedy for colds and flu.

Incorporating these antiviral herbs into your diet can provide powerful protection against respiratory viruses and boost your overall immune health.

Herbs to Combat Inflammation

Chronic inflammation can weaken the immune system and lead to various health issues. Certain herbs possess anti-inflammatory properties that can help reduce inflammation and support immune function.

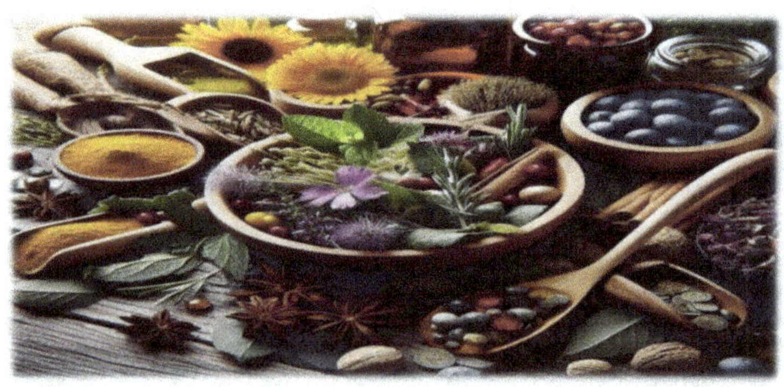

1. Turmeric

Properties: Curcumin, the active compound in turmeric, is a potent anti-inflammatory and antioxidant.

How to Use:

> **Golden Milk**: Mix turmeric powder with milk (dairy or plant-based), honey, and black pepper for enhanced absorption. Drink regularly.
> **Capsules**: Consider taking turmeric supplements for concentrated benefits.

Benefits: Turmeric helps to lower inflammation throughout the body, supporting immune function and overall health.

2. Ginger

Properties: Ginger contains gingerol, a compound known for its anti-inflammatory effects.

How to Use:

> **Tea**: Brew fresh ginger tea by steeping sliced ginger in hot water for 10-15 minutes. Add honey or lemon for flavor.
> **Powder**: Incorporate ginger powder into smoothies, soups, or stir-fries.

Benefits: Ginger not only reduces inflammation but also enhances circulation and promotes overall immune health.

3. Boswellia

Properties: Boswellia, or frankincense, has been used for centuries in traditional medicine for its anti-inflammatory properties.

How to Use:

> **Supplement**: Take boswellia extract in capsule form according to package directions.
> **Tea**: Brew boswellia tea using powdered resin.

Benefits: Boswellia helps to reduce inflammation in the body, supporting the immune system and relieving joint pain.

By incorporating these anti-inflammatory herbs into your diet, you can help reduce inflammation and bolster your immune health.

Adaptogens for Immune Balance

Adaptogens are herbs that help the body adapt to stress and maintain balance in the immune system. These herbs can enhance resilience and support overall health.

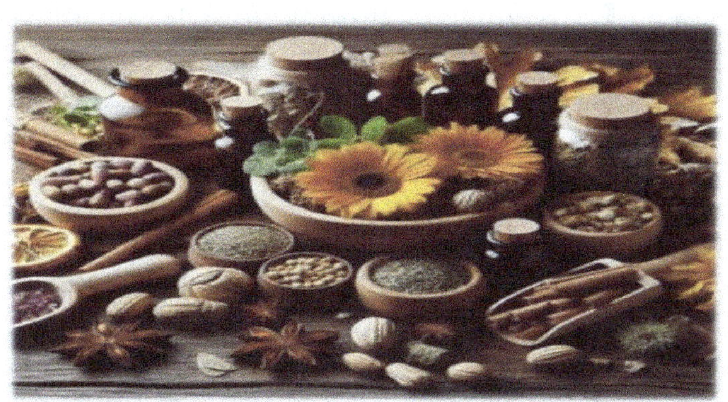

1. Astragalus

Properties: Astragalus is known for its immune-boosting and adaptogenic properties.

How to Use:

> **Tea**: Steep dried astragalus root in hot water for 10-15 minutes. Drink daily for immune support.
> **Tincture**: Use astragalus tincture as directed for added benefits.

Benefits: Astragalus enhances the immune response and helps the body adapt to stressors, promoting long-term health.

2. Ashwagandha

Properties: Ashwagandha is a well-known adaptogen that reduces stress and supports immune function.

How to Use:

- **Powder**: Mix ashwagandha powder into smoothies, warm milk, or oatmeal.
- **Capsules**: Take ashwagandha supplements according to the recommended dosage.

Benefits: Ashwagandha helps regulate immune responses and promotes overall well-being, especially during stressful times.

3. Rhodiola

Properties: Rhodiola is another powerful adaptogen known for its ability to enhance physical and mental resilience.

How to Use:

- **Tea**: Brew rhodiola root in hot water for a calming tea.
- **Capsules**: Take rhodiola supplements as directed.

Benefits: Rhodiola helps reduce fatigue and stress while supporting immune function.

Integrating these adaptogenic herbs into your daily routine can help balance your immune system and improve your body's resilience to stressors.

Herbal Antibiotics:

Understanding the Role of Goldenseal, Garlic, and Other Natural Antibiotics

Herbal antibiotics can offer natural alternatives to conventional antibiotics for combating infections. Understanding their roles can help you make informed choices for immune support.

1. Goldenseal

Properties: Goldenseal contains berberine, which has antimicrobial properties.

How to Use:

- ➢ **Tincture**: Take goldenseal tincture as directed for immune support.
- ➢ **Tea**: Brew goldenseal tea using dried root.

Benefits: Goldenseal is effective against various infections, especially those affecting the respiratory and digestive systems.

2. Garlic

Properties: As previously discussed, garlic possesses strong antimicrobial and immune-boosting properties.

How to Use:

> **Raw**: Crush and consume raw garlic for maximum benefits.
> **Supplement**: Take garlic capsules for a concentrated dose.

Benefits: Garlic helps fight infections, supports immune function, and can help lower blood pressure.

3. Oregano Oil

Properties: Oregano oil is rich in carvacrol and thymol, making it a potent natural antibiotic.

How to Use:

> **Oil**: Use diluted oregano oil for topical applications or take as a supplement.
> **Capsules**: Consider taking oregano oil capsules for internal use.

Benefits: Oregano oil has been shown to fight a variety of bacterial infections and support immune health.

Incorporating these herbal antibiotics into your health regimen can offer additional protection against infections while supporting your immune system.

Preventative Herbal Strategies:

Incorporating Immune-Boosting Herbs into Daily Life

Prevention is key when it comes to maintaining a robust immune system. Here are some actionable strategies to incorporate immune-boosting herbs into your daily routine:

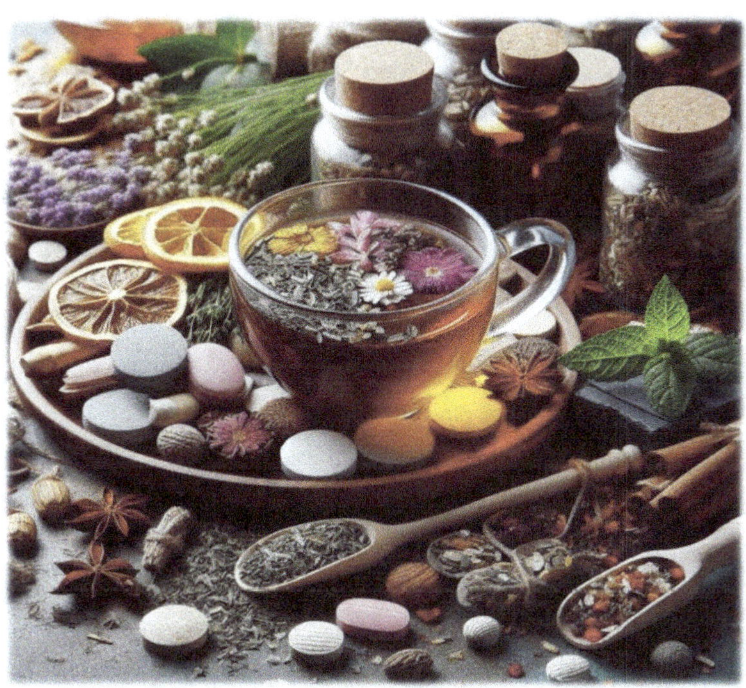

1. Daily Herbal Teas

➤ Start your day with a cup of herbal tea featuring immune-supporting herbs like echinacea, ginger, or chamomile. This can help kickstart your immune system each morning.

2. Smoothies and Soups

➤ Add herbs like turmeric, garlic, or ashwagandha to your smoothies or soups for a health boost. This not only enhances flavor but also increases your nutrient intake.

3. Supplementation

➤ Consider herbal supplements, especially during cold and flu season, to support your immune system proactively. Choose high-quality products from reputable sources.

4. Cooking with Herbs

➤ Incorporate fresh herbs like oregano, thyme, and basil into your cooking. They not only add flavor but also provide numerous health benefits.

Conclusion

Herbs for immune system support offer a natural and effective way to bolster your body's defenses. From the powerful effects of echinacea and elderberry to the antiviral properties of oregano and garlic, incorporating these herbs into your daily routine can enhance your overall health.

Additionally, understanding the roles of anti-inflammatory herbs, adaptogens, and natural antibiotics allows you to make informed choices for your immune health. By embracing herbal medicine and adopting preventative strategies, you can cultivate a resilient immune system and foster long-term wellness.

Remember to listen to your body, consult with a healthcare provider when necessary, and enjoy the journey of exploring the world of herbal remedies!

Chapter 06
Natural Remedies for Stress, Anxiety, and Sleep

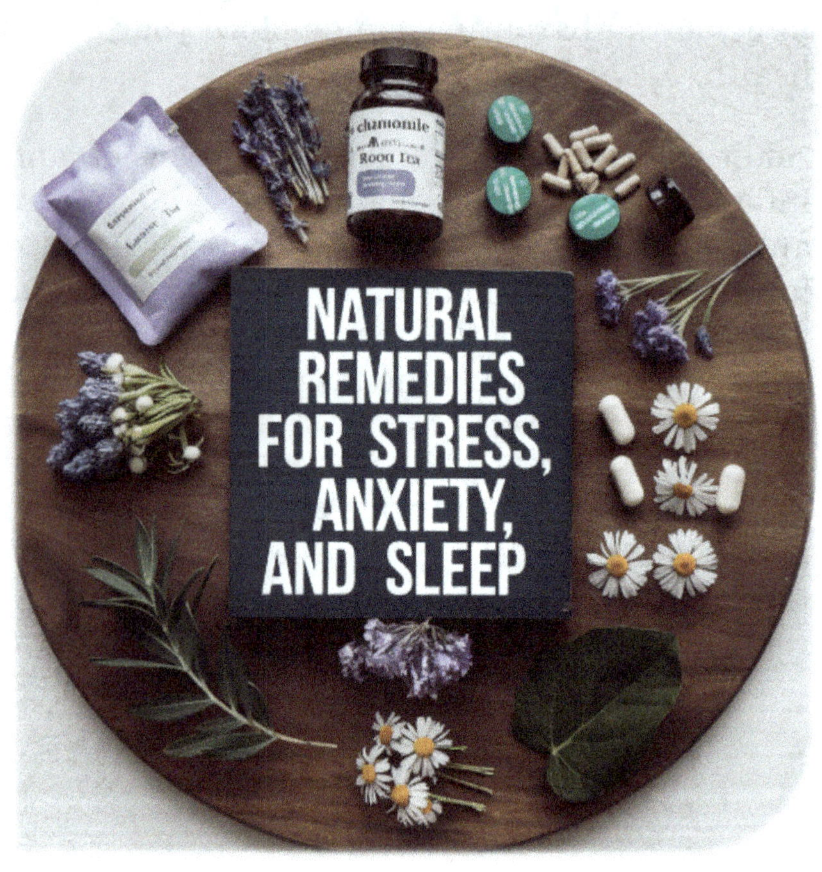

In our fast-paced world, stress and anxiety have become common experiences that can significantly impact our mental and physical health. Fortunately, nature offers a wealth of herbal remedies to help manage these challenges and promote restful sleep. In this chapter, we will explore various herbs that can help soothe stress, enhance mental clarity, and foster better sleep quality, along with actionable strategies to incorporate them into your daily routine.

Calming Herbs for Daily Stress

For everyday stress and anxiety, certain herbs can provide immediate relief and promote a sense of calm. Here are three of the most effective calming herbs:

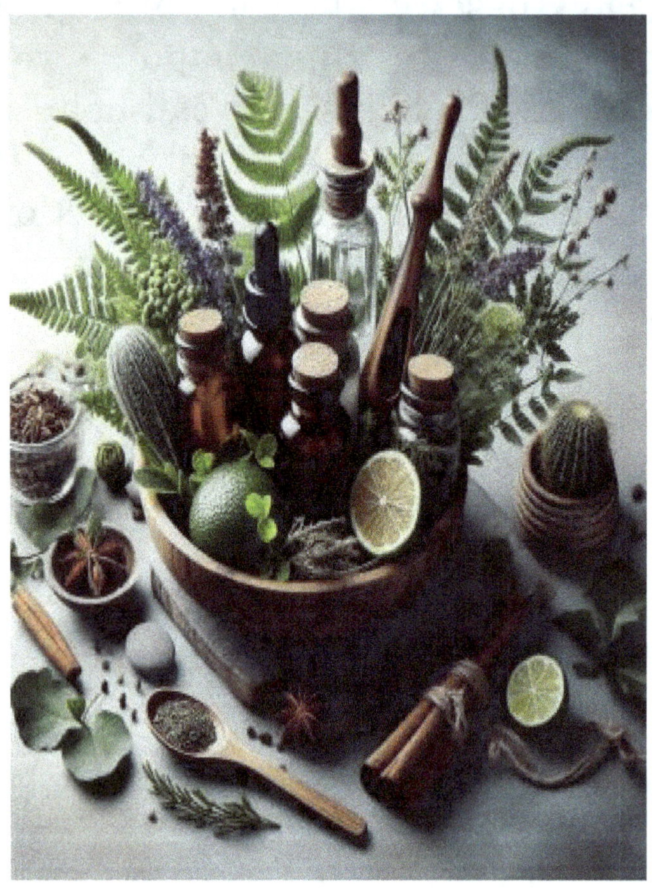

1. Chamomile

Properties: Chamomile is renowned for its soothing properties and is often used to alleviate anxiety and promote relaxation.

How to Use:

- ➢ **Tea**: Brew a cup of chamomile tea by steeping 1-2 teaspoons of dried flowers in hot water for 5-10 minutes. Drink it in the evening to unwind before bedtime.
- ➢ **Essential Oil**: Use chamomile essential oil in a diffuser or apply it topically (diluted) to promote relaxation.

Benefits: Chamomile has mild sedative effects, helping to reduce anxiety and improve sleep quality.

2. Lemon Balm

Properties: Lemon balm is a member of the mint family and is known for its calming effects on the nervous system.

How to Use:

- ➢ **Tea**: Prepare lemon balm tea by steeping fresh or dried leaves in hot water for 10 minutes. Consume it throughout the day as needed.
- ➢ **Tincture**: Use lemon balm tincture to promote relaxation during stressful situations.

Benefits: Lemon balm can reduce anxiety, improve mood, and promote a sense of calm.

3. Passionflower

Properties: Passionflower has been traditionally used to treat anxiety and insomnia due to its calming effects.

How to Use:

- **Tea**: Brew passionflower tea by steeping the dried leaves and flowers in hot water for 10-15 minutes. Enjoy before bed for optimal effects.
- **Capsules**: Take passionflower capsules as directed for additional support

Benefits: Passionflower helps increase the production of gamma-aminobutyric acid (GABA), a neurotransmitter that promotes relaxation and reduces anxiety.

Incorporating these calming herbs into your daily routine can provide effective relief from everyday stressors and promote a sense of well-being.

Adaptogens to Build Resilience

Adaptogens are herbs that help the body adapt to stress and maintain balance. These herbs can enhance resilience and support overall mental health.

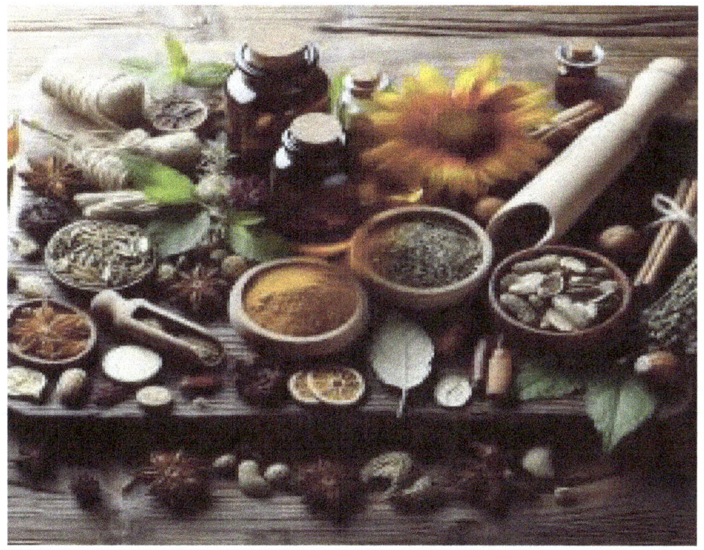

1. Ashwagandha

Properties: Ashwagandha is a powerful adaptogen known for its ability to combat stress and anxiety.

How to Use:

- **Powder**: Mix ashwagandha powder into smoothies, warm milk, or oatmeal.
- **Capsules**: Take ashwagandha supplements according to the recommended dosage.

Benefits: Ashwagandha lowers cortisol levels and promotes relaxation, helping the body adapt to stressors effectively.

2. Holy Basil (Tulsi)

Properties: Holy basil is revered in Ayurvedic medicine for its stress-relieving properties and ability to balance the mind and body.

How to Use:

➢ **Tea**: Brew holy basil tea using fresh or dried leaves for a refreshing drink that calms the mind.
➢ **Extract**: Take holy basil extract or capsules as directed.

Benefits: Holy basil helps reduce stress, improve mental clarity, and enhance overall well-being.

3. Rhodiola

Properties: Rhodiola is an adaptogen known for its ability to enhance energy, stamina, and mental clarity while reducing fatigue.

How to Use:

➢ **Tea**: Brew rhodiola tea from dried root for a calming yet energizing beverage.
➢ **Capsules**: Take rhodiola supplements according to the recommended dosage.

Benefits: Rhodiola helps improve mood, enhance cognitive function, and promote resilience against stress.

By integrating these adaptogenic herbs into your routine, you can build resilience to stress and support your overall mental health.

Herbal Sleep Aids

For those struggling with sleep issues, certain herbs can promote relaxation and improve sleep quality. Here are some effective herbal sleep aids:

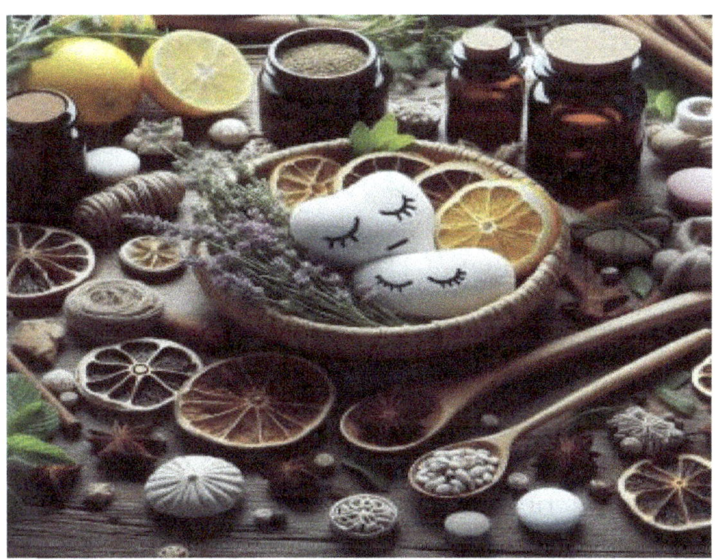

1. Valerian Root

Properties: Valerian root has been used for centuries as a natural remedy for insomnia and anxiety.

How to Use:

➢ **Tea**: Brew valerian root tea by steeping 1-2 teaspoons of dried root in hot water for 10-15 minutes. Drink 30 minutes to an hour before bedtime.
➢ **Tincture**: Take valerian tincture as directed for quick relief from insomnia.

Benefits: Valerian root promotes deeper sleep and reduces the time it takes to fall asleep.

2. California Poppy

Properties: California poppy is known for its calming effects and is often used to treat insomnia and anxiety.

How to Use:

➢ **Tea**: Brew California poppy tea by steeping dried flowers in hot water for 10-15 minutes before bedtime.
➢ **Tincture**: Use California poppy tincture for fast-acting support.

Benefits: California poppy helps improve sleep quality without the grogginess associated with some sleep medications.

3. Skullcap

Properties: Skullcap is an herbal remedy for anxiety and insomnia, promoting relaxation and restful sleep.

How to Use:

> **Tea**: Steep dried skullcap leaves in hot water for 10 minutes. Enjoy before bedtime to encourage relaxation.
> **Capsules**: Take skullcap capsules as needed for anxiety relief.

Benefits: Skullcap helps calm the mind, making it easier to fall asleep and stay asleep.

Incorporating these herbal sleep aids into your nighttime routine can help you achieve restful sleep and improve overall well-being.

Herbs for Mental Clarity and Focus

Certain herbs can enhance cognitive function, improve mental clarity, and support focus, making them beneficial for those facing stress or anxiety. Here are some powerful cognitive-supporting herbs:

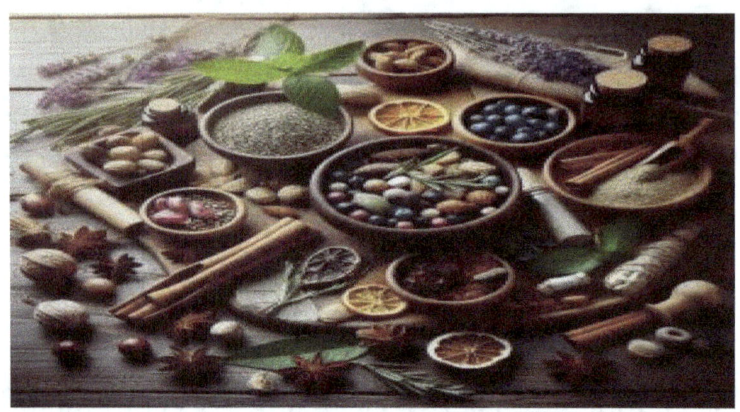

1. Ginkgo Biloba

Properties: Ginkgo biloba is well-known for its ability to improve memory and cognitive function.

How to Use:

> **Extract**: Take ginkgo extract or capsules as directed for enhanced cognitive support.
> **Tea**: Brew ginkgo tea using dried leaves for a refreshing beverage that supports focus.

Benefits: Ginkgo biloba enhances blood circulation to the brain, promoting better mental clarity and focus.

2. Gotu Kola

Properties: Gotu kola is an adaptogen that supports mental clarity and cognitive function.

How to Use:

> **Tea**: Brew gotu kola tea by steeping dried leaves in hot water for 10 minutes. Drink for improved focus and clarity.
> **Capsules**: Take gotu kola capsules as needed for cognitive support.

Benefits: Gotu kola enhances memory and concentration, making it a valuable herb for studying or working.

3. Bacopa Monnieri

Properties: Bacopa is an ancient herb used in Ayurvedic medicine to enhance memory and cognitive function.

How to Use:

> **Powder**: Mix bacopa powder into smoothies or warm milk.
> **Capsules**: Take bacopa supplements as directed for cognitive enhancement.

Benefits: Bacopa improves memory retention and supports overall cognitive health, particularly under stress.

Incorporating these herbs into your daily routine can help improve mental clarity and support cognitive function, particularly in times of stress.

Balancing Mood with Herbal Remedies

Mild to moderate depression can be effectively managed with certain herbs that help balance mood and support emotional well-being. Here are two herbs known for their mood-enhancing properties:

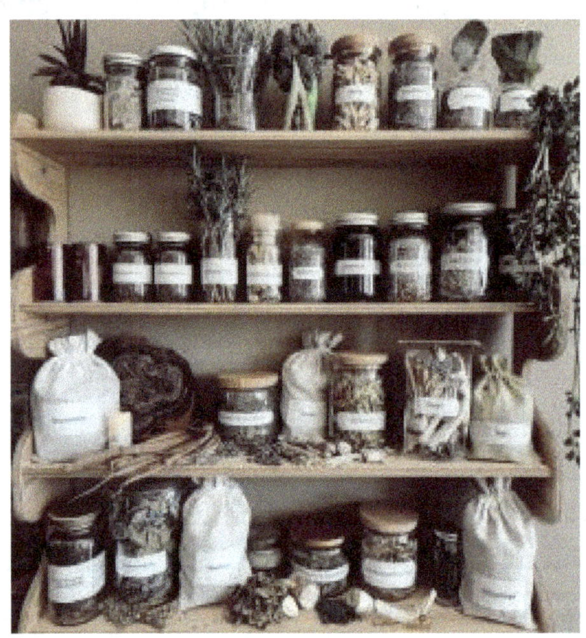

1. St. John's Wort

Properties: St. John's Wort is a well-researched herb for alleviating symptoms of mild to moderate depression.

How to Use:

- ➤ **Tea**: Brew St. John's Wort tea by steeping dried flowers in hot water for 10 minutes. Drink daily for mood support.
- ➤ **Capsules**: Take St. John's Wort capsules as directed for concentrated benefits.

Benefits: St. John's Wort works by increasing serotonin levels in the brain, which can improve mood and reduce anxiety.

2. Saffron

Properties: Saffron is a spice with mood-enhancing properties that can help alleviate symptoms of depression.

How to Use:

- ➤ **Tea**: Steep saffron threads in hot water to make a fragrant tea. Enjoy it daily for mood support.
- ➤ **Culinary Use**: Add saffron to your cooking to enhance flavor and benefit mood.

Benefits: Saffron has been shown to improve mood and reduce feelings of sadness, making it a delightful addition to your herbal regimen.

Integrating these mood-balancing herbs into your routine can support emotional well-being and foster a more positive outlook.

Creating a Stress-Relief Herbal Routine

To effectively manage stress, anxiety, and sleep disturbances, it's important to create a personalized herbal routine that works for you. Here are some actionable steps to design your stress-relief regimen:

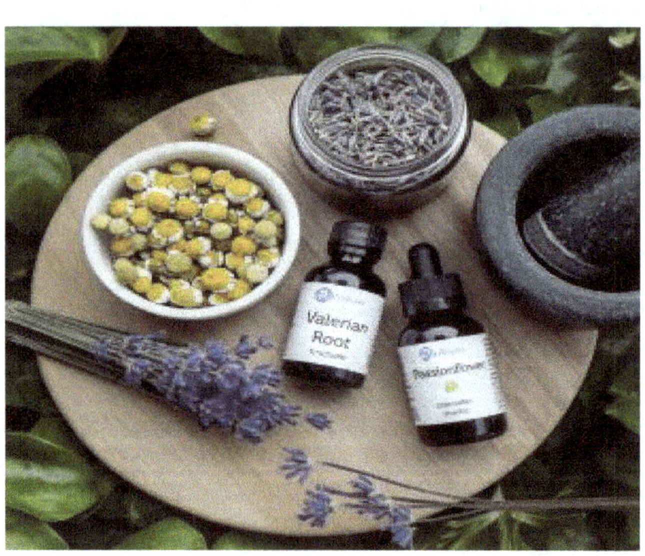

1. Assess Your Needs

> Identify the specific areas you want to address: daily stress, anxiety, sleep issues, or mood balance.

2. Choose Your Herbs

> Select 2-3 herbs from each category (calming, adaptogenic, sleep aids, cognitive support, and mood balancers) that resonate with you.

3. Create a Schedule

> Plan when you will take your herbs. Consider incorporating teas into your morning routine, tinctures during stressful moments, and calming herbs in the evening.

4. Make It Enjoyabl

> Find ways to enjoy your herbal remedies. Experiment with different tea blends, herbal syrups, or cooking with fresh herbs to keep your routine engaging.

5. Listen to Your Body

> Pay attention to how your body responds to different herbs and adjust your regimen accordingly. Consult with a healthcare professional if you experience any adverse effects.

6. Incorporate Mindfulness

> Combine your herbal routine with mindfulness practices, such as meditation or deep-breathing exercises, to enhance relaxation and stress relief.

By designing a personalized stress-relief herbal routine, you can effectively manage stress, enhance mental clarity, and promote better sleep.

Conclusion

The world of herbal remedies offers a natural and effective way to manage stress, anxiety, and sleep disturbances. From calming herbs like chamomile and passionflower to powerful adaptogens such as ashwagandha and rhodiola, there are numerous options to support your mental well-being.

By creating a personalized herbal routine that fits your unique needs, you can cultivate resilience against stress and enhance your overall quality of life. Remember, the journey toward well-being is a personal one, and incorporating herbal remedies can be a valuable step toward a healthier, more balanced life

Part 2:
Advanced Herbal Practices and Holistic Health

Chapter 07
Detoxifying and Cleansing with Herbs

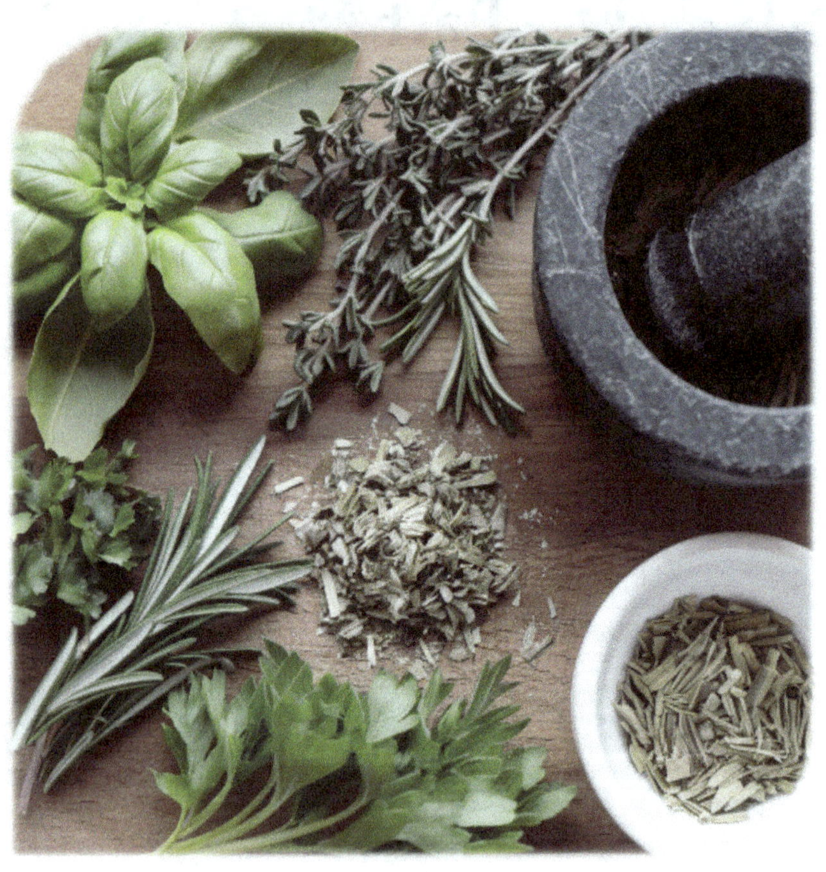

Detoxification is a vital aspect of maintaining overall health, allowing our bodies to eliminate toxins and promote optimal function. Herbal remedies have been used for centuries to support detoxification processes naturally. This chapter explores various herbs that assist in cleansing the body, with a focus on liver, kidney, lymphatic system, colon, and skin detoxification. We will also discuss how to build a seasonal herbal detox program to enhance your well-being throughout the year.

Liver Cleansing with Herbs

The liver is a key organ in the body's detoxification process, filtering toxins and metabolizing substances. Certain herbs can support liver function and promote its natural detoxification capabilities.

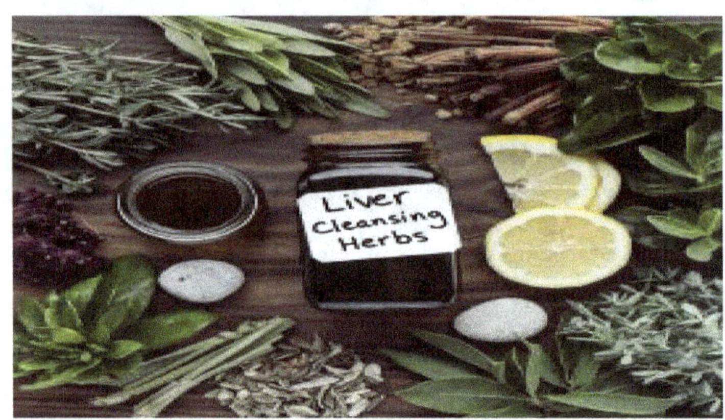

1. Milk Thistle

Properties: Milk thistle contains silymarin, a compound known for its protective effects on liver cells.

How to Use:

➢ **Capsules**: Take milk thistle capsules as directed, typically in dosages of 140–420 mg daily.
➢ **Tea**: Brew milk thistle tea from the seeds for a gentle liver tonic.

Benefits: Milk thistle promotes liver regeneration and protects against damage from toxins, alcohol, and medications.

2. Dandelion Root

Properties: Dandelion root is a bitter herb that stimulates bile production, enhancing liver function.

How to Use:

> **Tea**: Steep dried dandelion root in boiling water for 10-15 minutes. Drink this tea to stimulate digestion and liver function.
> **Tincture**: Take dandelion tincture for a concentrated dose.

Benefits: Dandelion root aids digestion and detoxification, promoting healthy liver function.

3. Artichoke

Properties: Artichoke leaves contain czarina, which supports bile production and liver health.

How to Use:

> **Tea**: Brew artichoke leaf tea to promote liver function.
> **Supplements**: Take artichoke extract or capsules as directed.

Benefits: Artichoke aids in detoxification and improves fat metabolism, supporting liver health.

Incorporating these herbs into your diet can help maintain optimal liver function and enhance your body's detoxification abilities.

Herbs to Support Kidney Health

The kidneys play a crucial role in filtering waste and regulating fluid balance. Supporting kidney health through herbal remedies can enhance their detoxification functions.

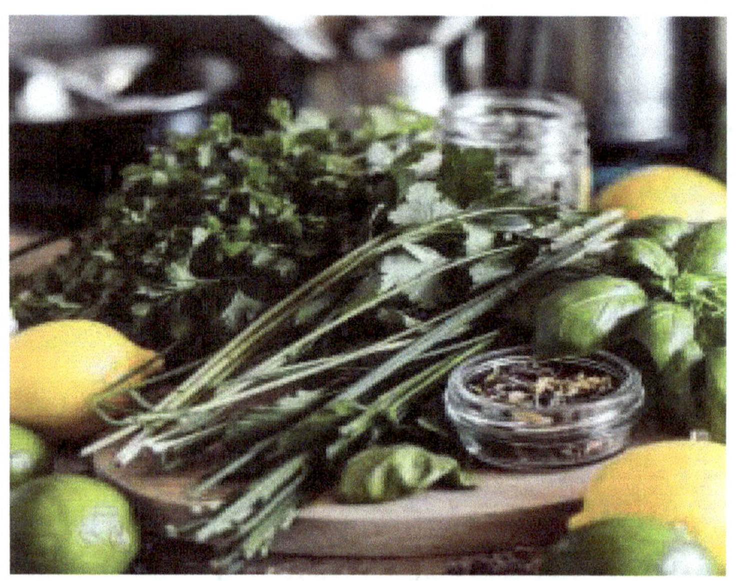

1. Nettle

Properties: Nettle is a diuretic herb that promotes kidney function and supports urinary health.

How to Use:

> **Tea**: Steep dried nettle leaves in hot water for 10-15 minutes. Drink this tea to promote kidney health.
> **Capsules**: Take nettle capsules as directed for added benefits.

Benefits: Nettle helps flush out toxins and supports kidney health by increasing urine output.

2. Parsley

Properties: Parsley is a natural diuretic that helps cleanse the kidneys and urinary tract.

How to Use:

> **Tea**: Brew parsley tea by steeping fresh or dried leaves in hot water for 10 minutes.
> **Culinary Use**: Add fresh parsley to salads, soups, or smoothies for daily kidney support.

Benefits: Parsley promotes healthy kidney function and helps eliminate waste products from the body.

3. Uva Ursi

Properties: Uva ursi, or bearberry, is known for its antimicrobial properties and its role in urinary health.

How to Use:

> **Tea**: Brew uva ursi tea by steeping dried leaves for 10-15 minutes. Consume as needed for urinary support.
> **Capsules**: Take uva ursi supplements as directed.

Benefits: Uva ursi helps reduce inflammation in the urinary tract and supports kidney function.

Incorporating these herbs into your wellness routine can enhance kidney health and promote detoxification.

Lymphatic System Detoxification

The lymphatic system plays a vital role in detoxification and immune function. Supporting lymphatic health through herbs can enhance the body's natural cleansing processes.

1. Red Clover

Properties: Red clover is a powerful lymphatic cleanser that promotes detoxification.

How to Use:

- ➤ **Tea**: Brew red clover tea by steeping dried flowers in hot water for 10-15 minutes. Drink daily for lymphatic support.
- ➤ **Tincture**: Use red clover tincture for concentrated benefits.

Benefits: Red clover supports lymphatic drainage and helps cleanse the body of toxins.

2. Cleavers

Properties: Cleavers are traditionally used to promote lymphatic function and drainage.

How to Use:

- ➤ **Tea**: Brew cleavers tea by steeping fresh or dried leaves in hot water for 10 minutes. Enjoy for lymphatic support.
- ➤ **Tincture**: Take cleavers tincture for enhanced effects.

Benefits: Cleavers help stimulate lymphatic flow, aiding in detoxification.

By incorporating these herbs into your routine, you can support lymphatic health and enhance your body's detoxification processes.

Herbal Colon Cleansing

A healthy colon is essential for overall health and detoxification. Several herbs can promote colon health and support regular elimination.

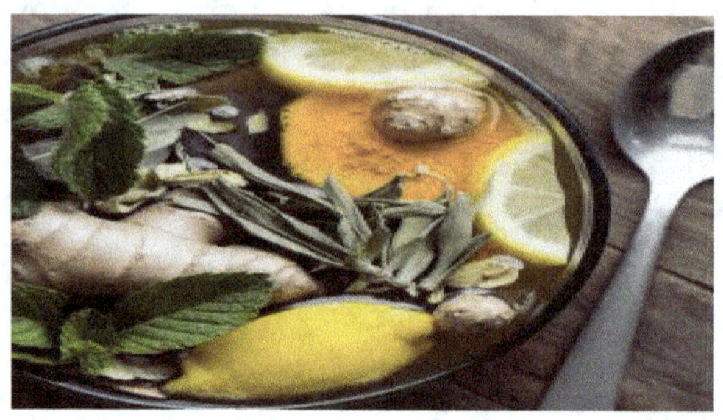

1. Psyllium

Properties: Psyllium is a soluble fiber that aids digestion and promotes regular bowel movements.

How to Use

- ➤ **Psyllium Husk**: Mix 1-2 tablespoons of psyllium husk with water or juice and drink immediately.
- ➤ **Supplements**: Take psyllium capsules as directed for digestive support.

Benefits: Psyllium promotes healthy digestion, aids in detoxification, and prevents constipation.

2. Flaxseed

Properties: Flaxseed is rich in fiber and omega-3 fatty acids, promoting digestive health.

How to Use:

> **Ground Flaxseed**: Add ground flaxseed to smoothies, oatmeal, or yogurt for digestive benefits.
> **Oil**: Use flaxseed oil in salad dressings for additional health benefits.

Benefits: Flaxseed supports regular bowel movements and aids in detoxification.

3. Aloe Vera

Properties: Aloe vera is known for its soothing properties and is often used to support digestive health.

How to Use:

> **Juice**: Drink aloe vera juice for digestive support and detoxification.
> **Gel**: Use aloe vera gel in smoothies or topical applications for skin health.

Benefits: Aloe vera promotes regularity and helps cleanse the colon.

Incorporating these herbs into your diet can support healthy digestion and promote regular elimination, enhancing your body's detoxification capabilities.

Supporting Skin Detoxification

The skin is the body's largest organ and plays a significant role in detoxification. Several herbs can help promote clear, healthy skin by supporting detoxification processes.

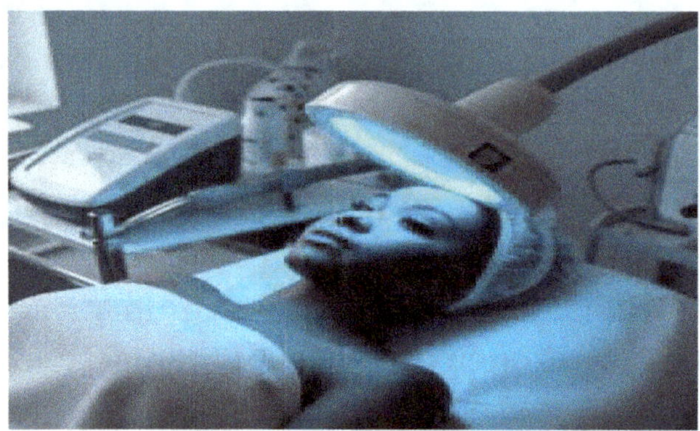

1. Burdock

Properties: Burdock is a traditional herbal remedy known for its blood-purifying properties.

How to Use:

➢ **Tea**: Brew burdock root tea by steeping dried root in hot water for 10-15 minutes.
➢ **Tincture**: Use burdock tincture for enhanced benefits.

Benefits: Burdock helps eliminate toxins from the bloodstream, promoting clear skin.

2. Echinacea

Properties: Echinacea is known for its immune-boosting properties and its ability to support skin health.

How to Use:

> **Tea**: Brew echinacea tea using dried flowers and leaves for immune and skin support.
> **Tincture**: Take echinacea tincture as directed for added benefits.

Benefits: Echinacea helps detoxify the skin and supports overall immune health.

3. Oregon Grape

Properties: Oregon grape contains berberine, which has antibacterial and antifungal properties, promoting healthy skin.

How to Use:

> **Tea**: Brew Oregon grape tea by steeping dried root in hot water.
> **Tincture**: Use Oregon grape tincture for enhanced skin benefits.

Benefits: Oregon grape supports skin detoxification and helps clear up skin issues.

By integrating these herbs into your skincare routine, you can promote healthy, clear skin while supporting your body's detoxification processes.

Building a Seasonal Herbal Detox Program

A seasonal herbal detox program can help you align your detoxification efforts with the changing seasons, enhancing your body's ability to cleanse and rejuvenate.

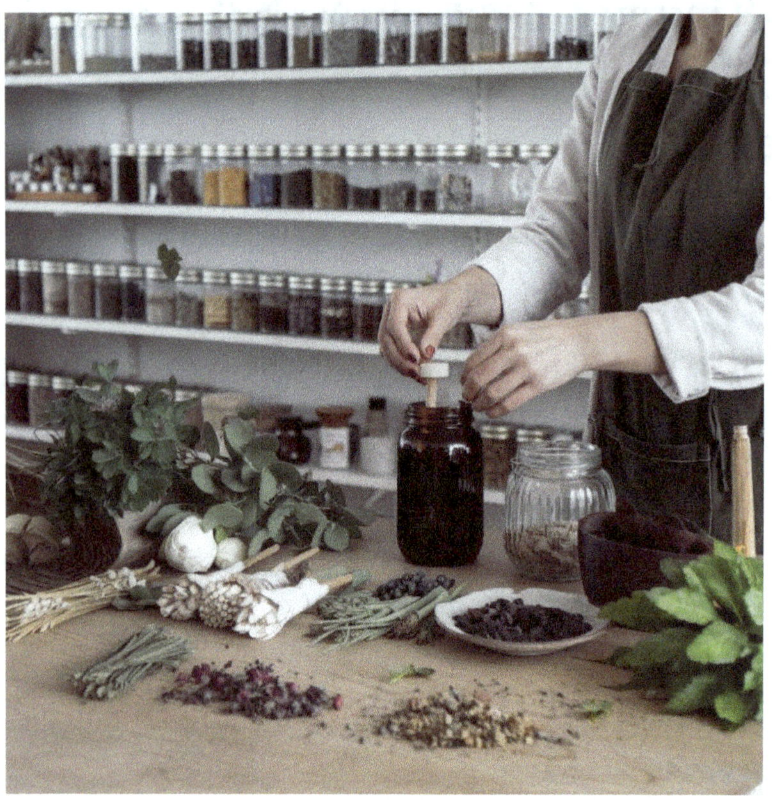

Here's how to create an effective seasonal detox program:

1. Spring Detox

- **Focus**: Emphasize liver and lymphatic health as your body naturally awakens from winter.
- **Herbs**: Incorporate milk thistle, dandelion root, and red clover.
- **Activities**: Engage in light exercise, outdoor walks, and increased hydration to support detoxification.

2. Summer Detox

- **Focus**: Support skin detoxification and hydration during the warm months.
- **Herbs**: Use burdock, echinacea, and peppermint to promote healthy skin and digestion.
- **Activities**: Prioritize outdoor activities, fresh fruits and vegetables, and plenty of water.

3. Fall Detox

- **Focus**: Prepare for winter by supporting lung and kidney health.
- **Herbs**: Include nettle, parsley, and mullein to strengthen the immune system.
- **Activities**: Incorporate warming foods and practices like meditation and gentle yoga.

4. Winter Detox

- **Focus**: Focus on internal detoxification and supporting immunity during colder months.

- ➢ **Herbs**: Use elderberry, garlic, and ginger for their immune-boosting properties.
- ➢ **Activities**: Emphasize warm teas, broth-based meals, and rest to enhance recovery.

Conclusion

Incorporating herbal remedies for detoxification can significantly enhance your body's ability to cleanse and rejuvenate. From supporting liver and kidney health to promoting skin detoxification, the right herbs can play a crucial role in your overall well-being. By building a seasonal herbal detox program, you can align your body's natural rhythms with your detoxification efforts, ensuring that you remain healthy and vibrant throughout the year.

With mindful practices and the appropriate herbal support, you can empower your body to eliminate toxins effectively and maintain optimal health, allowing you to thrive in your daily life.

Chapter 08
Herbal Support for Women's Health

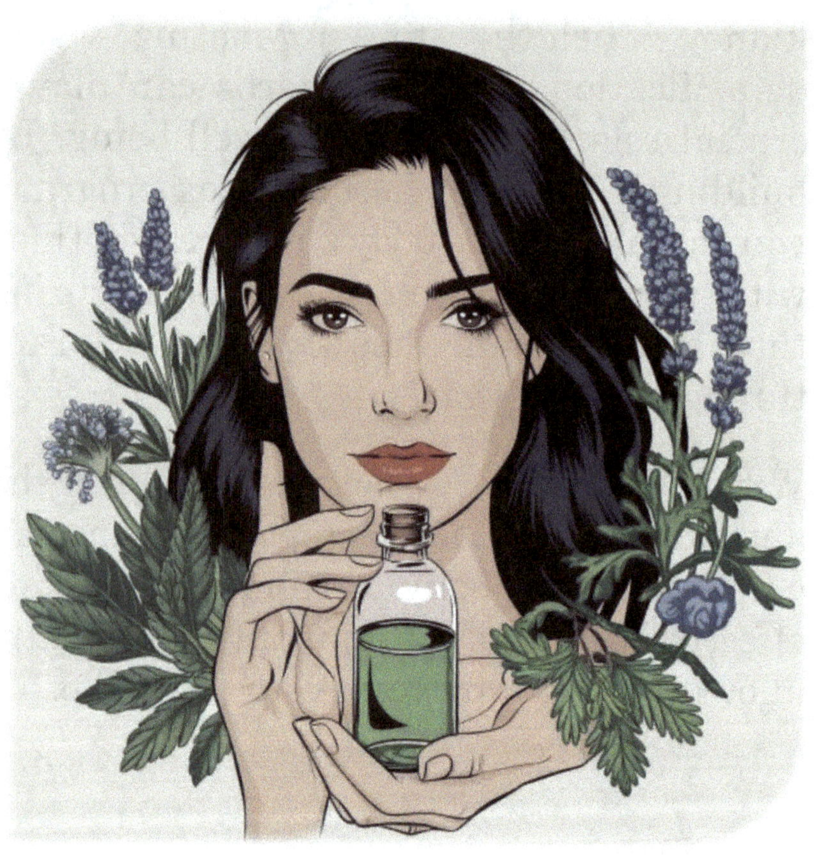

Women's health is a multifaceted area that encompasses various life stages, from menstruation to menopause and beyond. Herbal medicine offers a wealth of natural remedies that can support women through these transitions, addressing hormonal imbalances, reproductive health, and postpartum recovery. In this chapter, we will explore essential herbs for menstrual health, menopause, fertility, postpartum care, breast health, and hormonal balance, equipping you with knowledge to enhance your well-being naturally.

Herbs for Menstrual Health

Menstrual health is vital for overall well-being, and many women experience discomfort during their cycles. Certain herbs can help balance hormones and alleviate common menstrual issues.

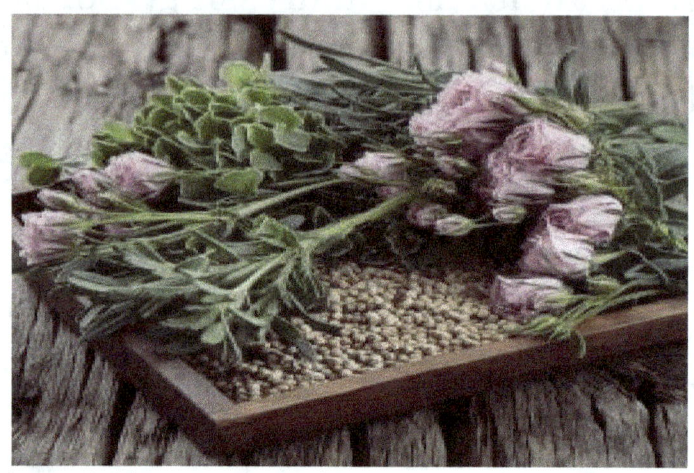

1. Vitex (Chaste Tree)

Properties: Vitex is known for its ability to regulate menstrual cycles and alleviate premenstrual syndrome (PMS) symptoms.

How to Use:

- ➤ **Tincture**: Take 20-40 drops of vitex tincture daily to support hormonal balance.
- ➤ **Capsules**: Follow the dosage instructions on vitex capsules, typically around 400-800 mg per day.

Benefits: Vitex may help reduce PMS symptoms, such as mood swings and breast tenderness, by balancing progesterone levels.

2. Black Cohosh

Properties: Black cohosh is traditionally used to alleviate menstrual discomfort and support hormonal health.

How to Use:

> **Tea**: Brew black cohosh tea by steeping the root in hot water for 10-15 minutes. Drink as needed for menstrual discomfort.
> **Capsules**: Follow the dosage instructions on black cohosh supplements, generally around 40-80 mg daily.

Benefits: Black cohosh can help ease cramps and regulate menstrual cycles.

3. Raspberry Leaf

Properties: Raspberry leaf is rich in vitamins and minerals that support menstrual health and tone the uterus.

How to Use:

> **Tea**: Brew raspberry leaf tea by steeping dried leaves for 10 minutes. Drink daily, especially during the luteal phase of your cycle.
> **Tincture**: Use raspberry leaf tincture for a concentrated dose.

Benefits: Raspberry leaf helps reduce menstrual pain and supports overall reproductive health.

Incorporating these herbs into your routine can help alleviate menstrual discomfort and support hormonal balance throughout your cycle.

Natural Remedies for Menopause

Menopause marks a significant transition in a woman's life, often accompanied by various symptoms such as hot flashes, mood swings, and sleep disturbances. Herbal remedies can provide natural support during this time.

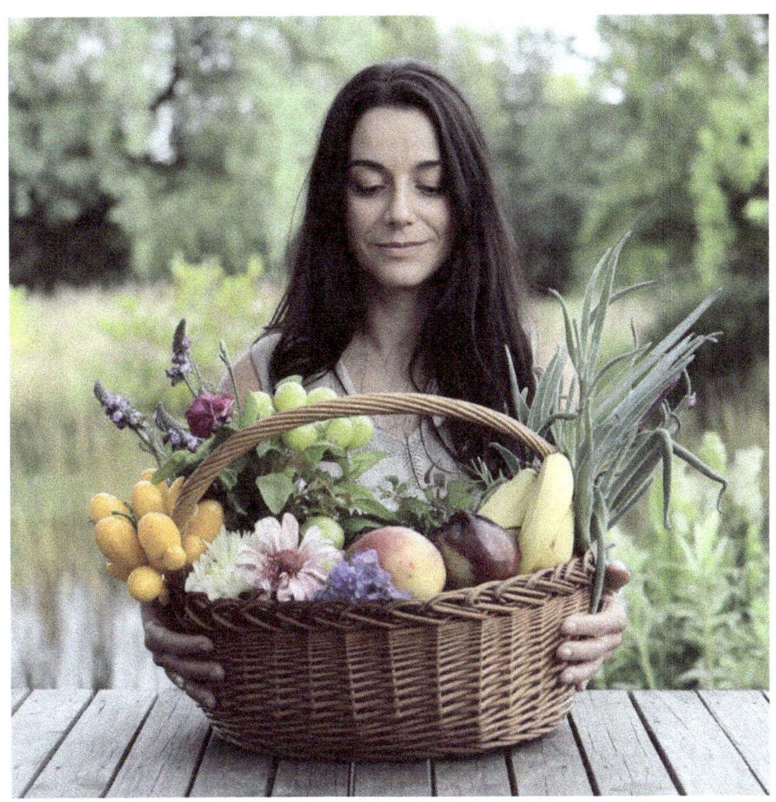

1. Red Clover

Properties: Red clover is rich in phytoestrogens, which can help balance hormones during menopause.

How to Use:

- ➤ **Tea**: Brew red clover tea by steeping dried flowers in hot water for 10-15 minutes. Enjoy daily for hormone support.
- ➤ **Tincture**: Take red clover tincture for a concentrated dose.

Benefits: Red clover can help reduce hot flashes and improve overall hormonal balance during menopause.

2. Dong Quai

Properties: Dong quai is known as "female ginseng" and is traditionally used to support women's reproductive health.

How to Use:

- ➤ **Tea**: Brew dong quai tea by steeping dried root in hot water. Drink this tea for hormonal support.
- ➤ **Capsules**: Follow dosage instructions on dong quai supplements, typically around 500-1,000 mg daily.

Benefits: Dong quai may help alleviate hot flashes and mood swings associated with menopause.

3. Sage

Properties: Sage has been used for centuries to reduce sweating and hot flashes.

How to Use:

➤ **Tea**: Brew sage tea by steeping fresh or dried leaves in hot water for 10 minutes. Drink as needed for hot flashes.

➤ **Tincture**: Use sage tincture for concentrated benefits.

Benefits: Sage can help regulate body temperature and reduce menopausal symptoms.

These herbs offer natural alternatives to manage menopausal symptoms, helping to ease the transition with greater comfort.

Fertility-Boosting Herbs

For women trying to conceive, certain herbs can support reproductive health and enhance fertility.

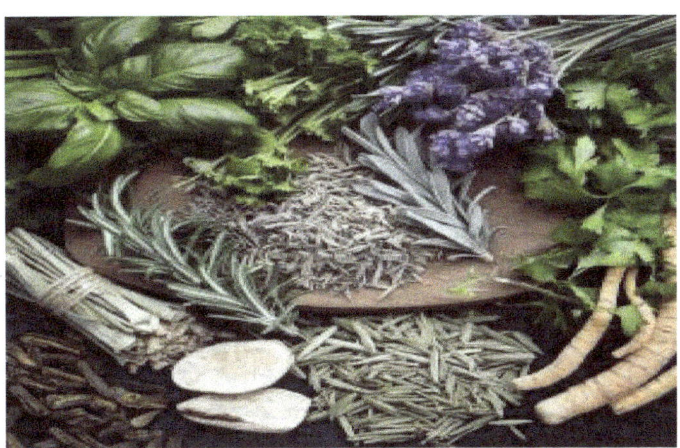

1. Maca

Properties: Maca is a nutrient-dense root that supports hormonal balance and reproductive health.

How to Use:

- ➤ **Powder**: Add 1-2 teaspoons of maca powder to smoothies, oatmeal, or baked goods for daily use.
- ➤ **Capsules**: Take maca capsules as directed, usually around 500-3,000 mg daily.

Benefits: Maca is known to enhance libido and improve hormonal balance, making it a valuable ally for those seeking to conceive.

2. Red Clover

Properties: In addition to its menstrual benefits, red clover supports reproductive health by providing essential nutrients.

How to Use:

- ➤ **Tea**: Brew red clover tea and drink daily to support fertility.
- ➤ **Tincture**: Take red clover tincture for a concentrated dose.

Benefits: Red clover's phytoestrogens can help regulate menstrual cycles and promote overall reproductive health.

3. Nettle

Properties: Nettle is rich in nutrients that support hormonal balance and overall reproductive health.

How to Use:

- ➤ **Tea**: Brew nettle leaf tea for daily consumption.
- ➤ **Capsules**: Take nettle capsules as directed.

Benefits: Nettle helps nourish the body, promoting healthy reproductive function.

Incorporating these herbs into your diet can provide essential support for women seeking to enhance their fertility naturally.

Postpartum Care with Herbs

After childbirth, women often face physical and emotional challenges. Certain herbs can provide nourishment and support during the postpartum period.

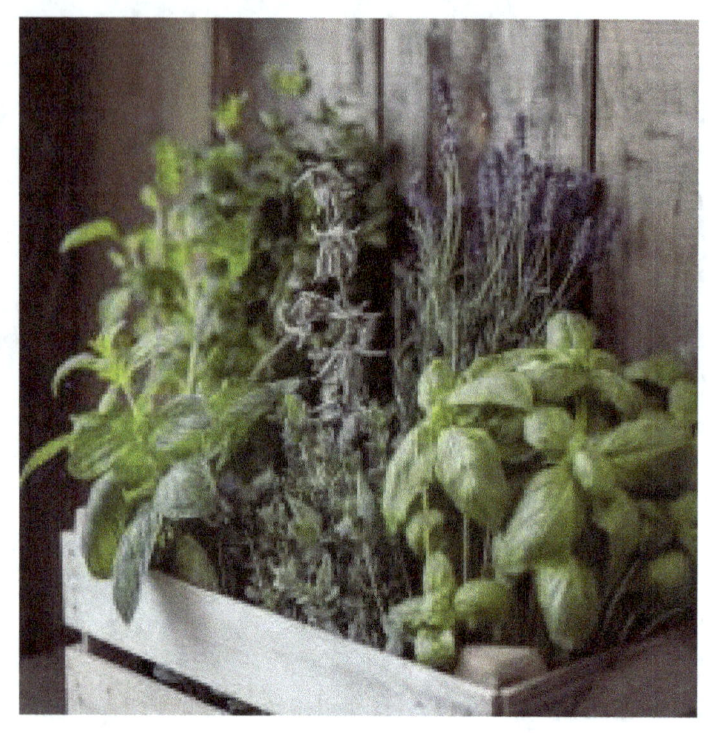

1. Shatavari

Properties: Shatavari is an adaptogenic herb known for its nourishing properties, particularly for women's reproductive health.

How to Use:

> **Powder**: Mix 1-2 teaspoons of shatavari powder into smoothies or warm milk.
> **Capsules**: Follow dosage instructions on shatavari supplements, typically around 500-1,000 mg daily.

Benefits: Shatavari helps balance hormones, supports lactation, and nourishes the body during the postpartum phase.

2. Motherwort

Properties: Motherwort is traditionally used to support emotional well-being and relieve anxiety.

How to Use:

> **Tea**: Brew motherwort tea by steeping dried leaves in hot water for 10-15 minutes. Drink as needed for emotional support.
> **Tincture**: Use motherwort tincture for concentrated effects.

Benefits: Motherwort can help ease postpartum anxiety and promote relaxation.

By incorporating these nourishing herbs, postpartum women can support their physical and emotional well-being during the recovery period.

Herbal Support for Breast Health

Breast health is an essential aspect of women's health, and several herbs can provide support for breast tissue and lymphatic function.

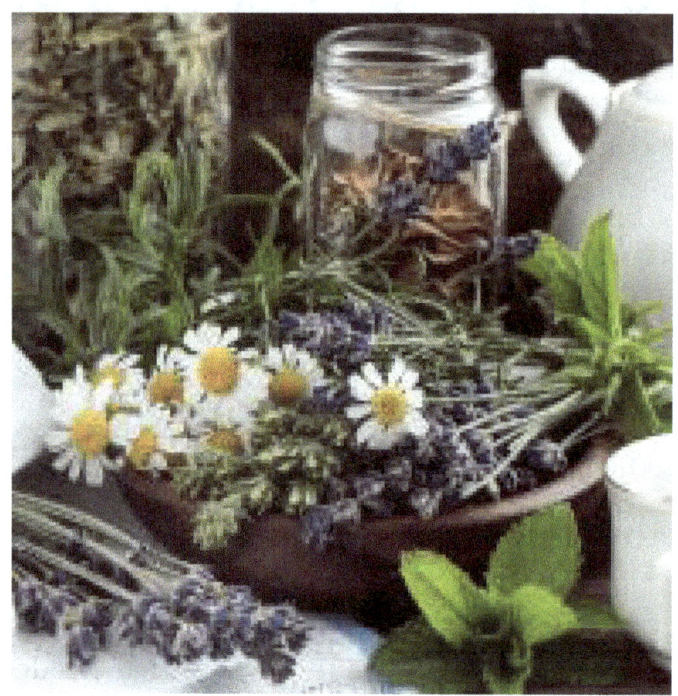

1. Calendula

Properties: Calendula is known for its anti-inflammatory properties and is often used to support breast health.

How to Use:

> **Infusion**: Make a calendula infusion by steeping dried flowers in oil for topical applications.
> **Tea**: Brew calendula tea for internal support.

Benefits: Calendula promotes lymphatic drainage and supports overall breast health.

2. Poke Root

Properties: Poke root is traditionally used for its ability to support lymphatic health.

How to Use:

> **Tincture**: Use poke root tincture carefully, as it is potent. Follow dosage instructions closely.
> **Topical Application**: Use poke root oil to massage the breast area for lymphatic support.

Benefits: Poke root aids in lymphatic drainage, promoting healthy breast tissue.

3. Red Clover

Properties: As previously mentioned, red clover supports breast health by providing phytoestrogens.

How to Use:

> **Tea**: Brew red clover tea for internal support.
> **Tincture**: Take red clover tincture for concentrated benefits.

Benefits: Red clover can help balance hormones and promote breast health.

These herbs can provide vital support for women's breast health, helping to maintain overall wellness.

Natural Remedies for Hormonal Balance

Hormonal imbalances can affect women at various stages of life. Certain herbs can help restore balance and support overall well-being.

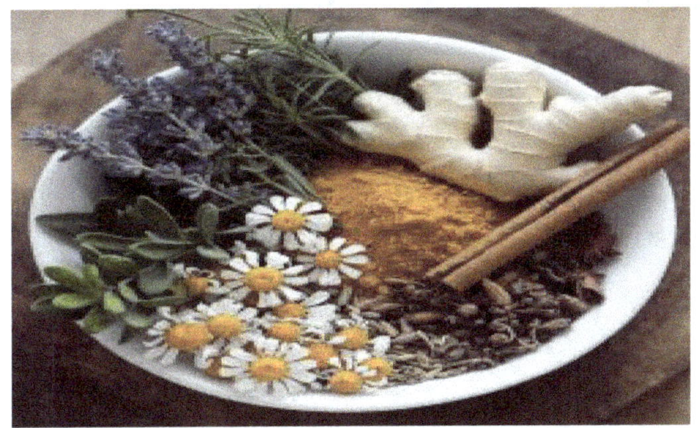

1. Ashwagandha

Properties: Ashwagandha is an adaptogen that helps reduce stress and support hormonal balance.

How to Use:

> **Powder**: Mix ashwagandha powder into smoothies or warm milk.
> **Capsules**: Follow dosage instructions for ashwagandha supplements, typically around 300-500 mg daily.

Benefits: Ashwagandha helps reduce cortisol levels, promoting hormonal balance and overall health.

2. Schisandra

Properties: Schisandra is another adaptogenic herb that supports adrenal function and hormonal balance.

How to Use:

> **Tincture**: Use schisandra tincture for concentrated benefits.
> **Tea**: Brew schisandra tea by steeping dried berries.

Benefits: Schisandra enhances the body's resilience to stress, supporting hormonal health.

Conclusion

Herbal support for women's health encompasses various aspects, from menstrual health to postpartum care. By incorporating the right herbs into your routine, you can address specific health concerns and promote overall well-being.

Whether you're seeking to balance hormones, enhance fertility, or support your body during menopause, these natural remedies provide effective solutions. Empower yourself with the knowledge and tools to harness the healing potential of herbs, and embrace a holistic approach to women's health that nurtures your body, mind, and spirit. Remember, as you explore these remedies, consult with a healthcare professional, especially when considering herbal supplements alongside other treatments. Your journey towards optimal health and wellness is uniquely yours, and the right herbal allies can make all the difference.

Chapter 09
Herbs for Skin and Hair Health

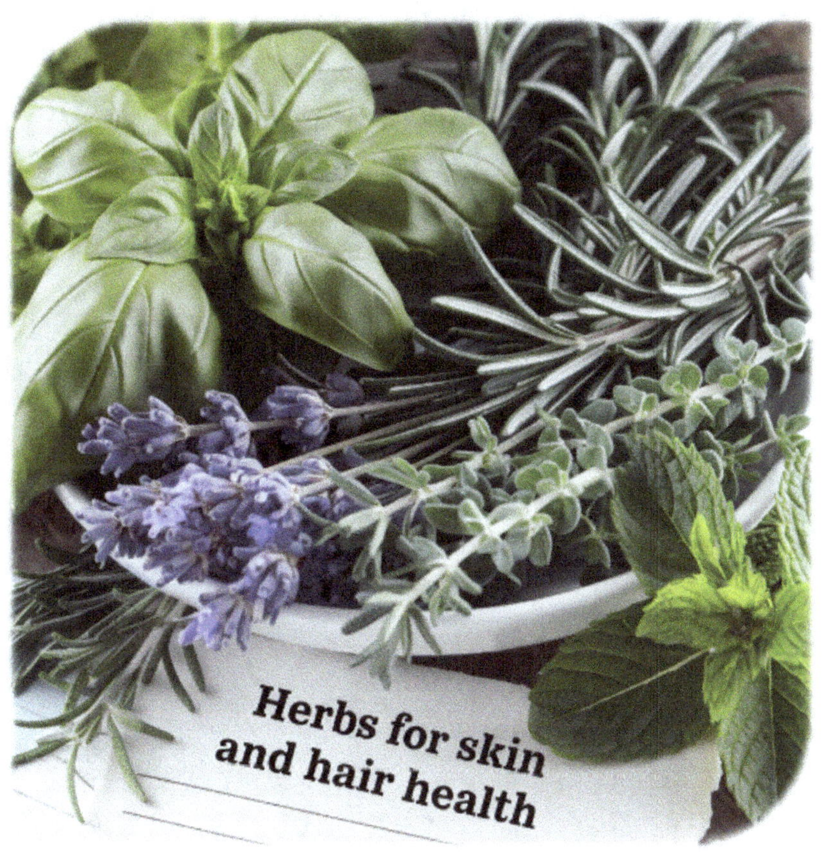

Our skin and hair are reflections of our overall health, often revealing the internal state of our bodies. As the body's largest organ, the skin protects against environmental factors while playing a crucial role in detoxification and overall appearance. Similarly, hair health is tied to nutrition, lifestyle, and emotional well-being. This chapter delves into how herbs can be powerful allies in achieving and maintaining radiant skin and luscious hair. From herbal infusions for hair growth to treatments for specific skin conditions, you'll discover practical, actionable remedies to enhance your beauty naturally.

Herbal Infusions for Hair Growth

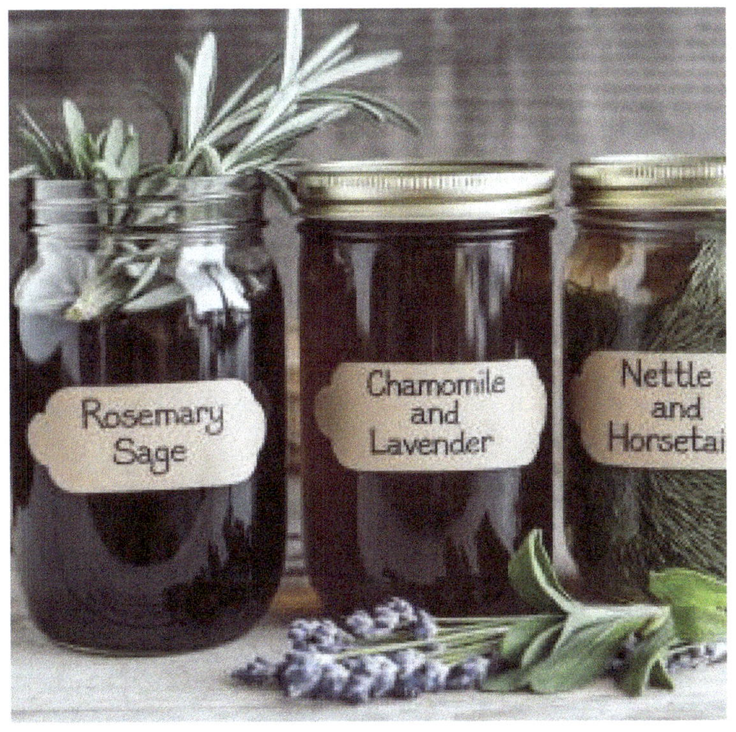

Healthy hair starts at the roots, and certain herbs can strengthen hair follicles, promote growth, and enhance shine.

1. Rosemary

Properties: Rosemary is well-known for stimulating hair follicles, increasing circulation to the scalp, and preventing hair loss.

How to Use:

1. **Infusion**: Brew rosemary tea by steeping fresh or dried rosemary leaves in boiling water for 10-15 minutes. Allow the infusion to cool, and use it as a rinse after shampooing to promote hair growth.
2. **Hair Oil**: Combine rosemary essential oil with a carrier oil (such as coconut or jojoba oil) and massage it into the scalp to stimulate hair growth.

Benefits: Regular use can lead to stronger hair, improved scalp health, and potential regrowth of thinning hair.

2. Nettle

Properties: Rich in vitamins A, C, K, and minerals like silica and iron, nettle supports overall hair health and growth.

How to Use:

> **Tea**: Brew nettle tea by steeping dried nettle leaves in hot water for 10-15 minutes. Drink this daily for optimal results.
> **Hair Rinse**: Use cooled nettle tea as a final rinse after washing your hair.

Benefits: Nettle helps nourish the scalp, promotes hair growth, and can reduce dandruff.

3. Horsetail

Properties: Horsetail contains silica, which is essential for healthy hair and skin.

How to Use:

> **Tea**: Brew horsetail tea by steeping dried horsetail in hot water. Drink regularly for benefits.
> **Hair Rinse**: Use horsetail tea as a hair rinse to strengthen hair and add shine.

Benefits: Strengthens hair strands, reduces breakage, and enhances overall hair health.

Incorporating these herbal infusions into your hair care routine can help promote healthier, stronger hair.

Treating Eczema and Psoriasis Naturally

Skin conditions like eczema and psoriasis can be uncomfortable and challenging to manage. Certain herbs possess anti-inflammatory, soothing, and healing properties that can provide relief.

1. Calendula

Properties: Known for its anti-inflammatory and healing properties, calendula can soothe irritated skin and promote healing.

How to Use:

> **Infused Oil**: Create a calendula-infused oil by steeping dried flowers in a carrier oil for 4-6 weeks. Use this oil to massage affected areas.
> **Salve**: Make a calendula salve by mixing infused oil with beeswax and applying it to inflamed skin.

Benefits: Helps reduce redness and irritation associated with eczema and psoriasis.

2. Chickweed

Properties: Chickweed has cooling and soothing properties, making it ideal for relieving itchy skin.

How to Use:

> **Salve**: Create a chickweed salve by infusing dried chickweed in a carrier oil, then adding beeswax. Apply to affected areas for relief.
> **Tea**: Drink chickweed tea to benefit from its anti-inflammatory properties internally.**Benefits**:

Alleviates itching and irritation, making it helpful for eczema and psoriasis sufferers.

3. Licorice Root

Properties: Licorice root contains glycyrrhizin, which has anti-inflammatory and immune-boosting properties.

How to Use:

➤ **Topical Application**: Create a paste using licorice root powder mixed with water or aloe vera gel. Apply it to inflamed skin.

➤ **Tea**: Drink licorice root tea to support skin health from the inside out.

Benefits: Licorice root helps reduce inflammation and redness associated with eczema and psoriasis.

By incorporating these herbs into your skincare routine, you can find natural relief from eczema and psoriasis symptoms.

Herbs for Acne-Prone Skin

Acne can be a source of frustration and insecurity for many. Luckily, certain herbs can help clear up blemishes, reduce inflammation, and promote a clearer complexion.

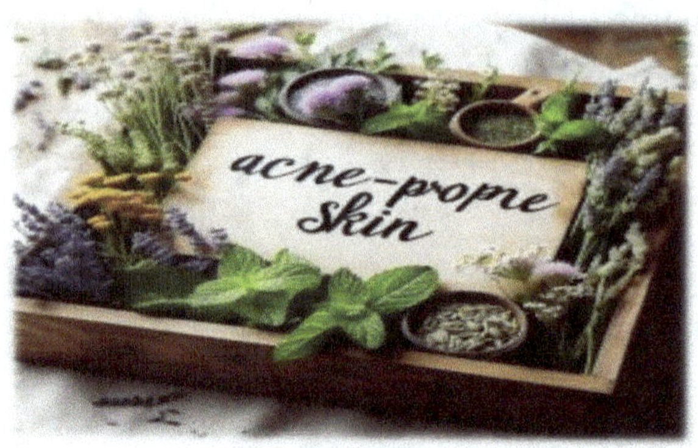

1. Burdock

Properties: Burdock root has detoxifying properties that can help cleanse the skin and reduce acne.

How to Use:

> **Tea**: Brew burdock root tea and drink it regularly to support internal detoxification.
> **Topical Application**: Create a paste from burdock root powder mixed with water and apply it to acne-prone areas.

Benefits: Helps purify the blood and can reduce the occurrence of acne breakouts.

2. Oregon Grape

Properties: Oregon grape contains berberine, which has antimicrobial properties effective against acne-causing bacteria.

How to Use:

➢ **Tea**: Brew Oregon grape tea and drink for skin-clearing benefits.
➢ **Tincture**: Apply Oregon grape tincture diluted with water to affected areas for targeted treatment.

Benefits: Reduces inflammation and promotes clearer skin.

3. Tea Tree Oil

Properties: Tea tree oil is well-known for its antibacterial and anti-inflammatory properties.

How to Use:

➢ **Topical Application**: Dilute tea tree oil with a carrier oil and apply it directly to acne spots.
➢ **Face Wash**: Add a few drops of tea tree oil to your regular face wash for added antibacterial benefits.

Benefits: Tea tree oil can significantly reduce the severity of acne and prevent future breakouts.

Incorporating these herbs into your skincare routine can help combat acne and promote a clearer, healthier complexion.

Soothing Inflammatory Skin Conditions

Sensitive skin can react to a variety of triggers, resulting in inflammation and irritation. Certain herbs can provide soothing relief for these conditions.

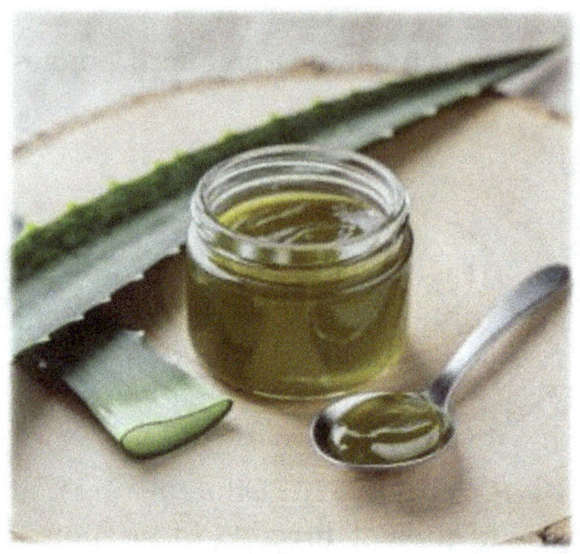

1. Aloe Vera

Properties: Aloe vera is renowned for its soothing and moisturizing properties, making it ideal for irritated skin.

How to Use:

> **Fresh Gel**: Apply fresh aloe vera gel directly from the plant to inflamed skin.
> **Infused Oil**: Create an aloe-infused oil by steeping aloe in a carrier oil for soothing effects.

Benefits: Aloe vera promotes healing, reduces redness, and provides moisture to the skin.

2. Chamomile

Properties: Chamomile has anti-inflammatory and calming effects that can soothe sensitive skin.

How to Use:

> **Tea**: Brew chamomile tea and use it as a compress on inflamed areas.
> **Topical Application**: Create a chamomile-infused oil for massage on sensitive areas.
> **Benefits**: Chamomile helps calm irritation and redness, making it beneficial for conditions like eczema and rosacea.

3. Lavender

Properties: Lavender possesses calming and anti-inflammatory properties, making it a great herb for sensitive skin.

How to Use:

> **Essential Oil**: Dilute lavender essential oil in a carrier oil and apply it to irritated skin.
> **Tea**: Brew lavender tea for internal calming effects.

Benefits: Lavender can help reduce inflammation and promote relaxation, aiding in skin recovery.

These soothing herbs can help calm inflammation and irritation, offering natural relief for sensitive skin.

Herbal Oils for Skin Rejuvenation

As we age, the skin requires additional nourishment to maintain its elasticity and youthfulness. Herbal oils can offer rejuvenating benefits to promote a healthy complexion.

1. Rosehip Oil

Properties: Rich in essential fatty acids and antioxidants, rosehip oil is excellent for skin rejuvenation.

How to Use:

> **Topical Application**: Apply rosehip oil directly to the skin after cleansing to hydrate and promote healing.
> **Face Serum**: Mix rosehip oil with a few drops of essential oil (like lavender) for a nourishing face serum.

Benefits: Rosehip oil helps reduce the appearance of scars, fine lines, and uneven skin tone.

2. Evening Primrose Oil

Properties: Evening primrose oil contains gamma-linolenic acid (GLA), which can help nourish and hydrate the skin.

How to Use:

- ➢ **Topical Application**: Apply evening primrose oil directly to dry or irritated skin.
- ➢ **Capsules**: Take evening primrose oil capsules as directed to support skin health from within.

Benefits: Helps improve skin elasticity and reduce signs of aging.

3. Sea Buckthorn Oil

Properties: Sea buckthorn oil is rich in vitamins A, C, and E, making it an excellent choice for skin rejuvenation.

How to Use:

- ➢ **Topical Application**: Apply sea buckthorn oil directly to the skin to hydrate and promote a healthy glow.
- ➢ **Face Mask**: Mix sea buckthorn oil with clay or honey for a rejuvenating face mask.

Benefits: Sea buckthorn oil supports skin regeneration, promoting a youthful appearance.

Incorporating these herbal oils into your skincare routine can significantly enhance skin health and rejuvenation.

Herbal Masks and Tonics:

DIY Treatments for Radiant Skin

Creating your own herbal masks and tonics can be an enjoyable and rewarding experience. Here are some simple recipes for DIY treatments that can nourish and rejuvenate your skin.

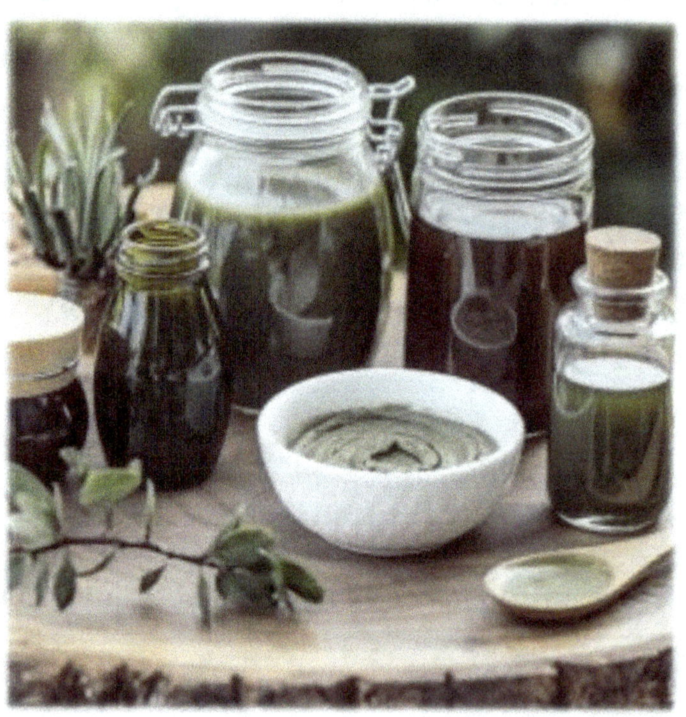

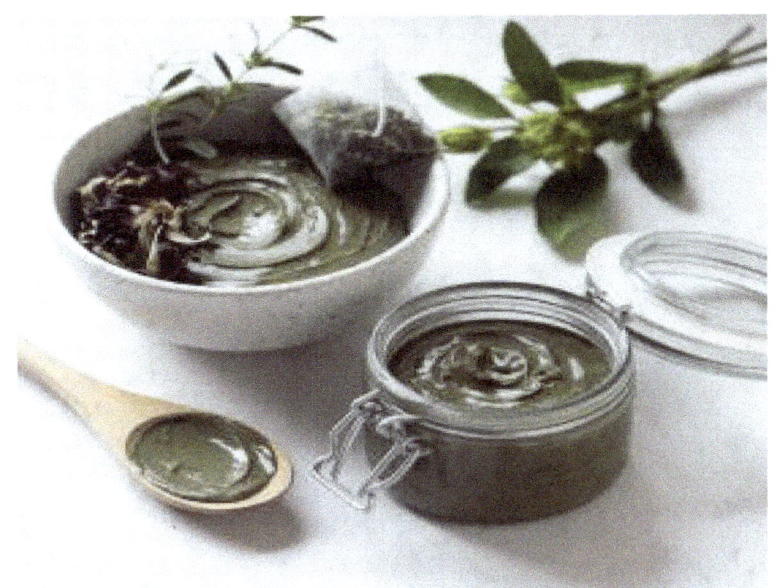

Herbal Face Mask for Hydration

Ingredients:

- ➤ 1 tablespoon honey
- ➤ 1 tablespoon yogurt
- ➤ 1 teaspoon rosehip oil
- ➤ 1 teaspoon chamomile tea (cooled)

Instructions:

- ➤ Mix all ingredients in a bowl until well combined.
- ➤ Apply to clean skin and leave on for 15-20 minutes.
- ➤ Rinse with warm water and pat dry.

Benefits: This mask provides hydration and nourishment, leaving your skin soft and glowing.

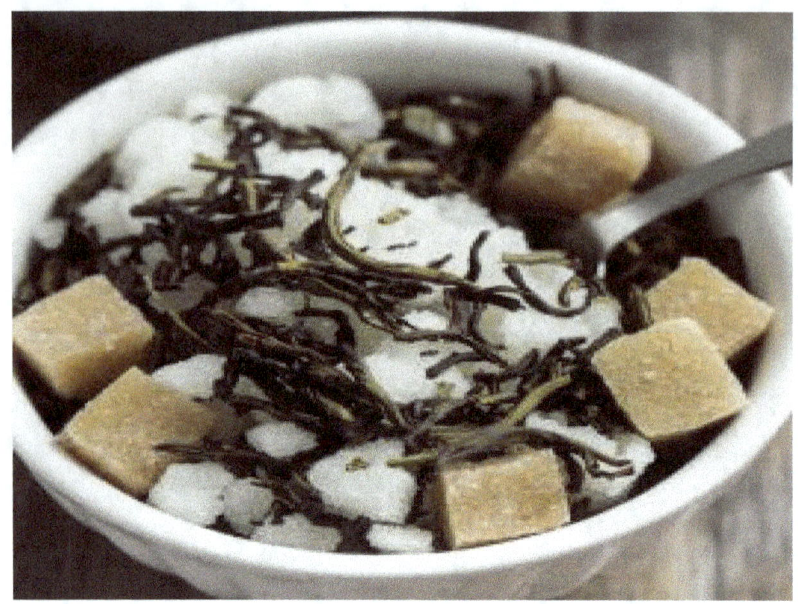

Exfoliating Herbal Scrub

Ingredients:

➢ 2 tablespoons sugar or salt
➢ 1 tablespoon coconut oil
➢ 1 teaspoon lavender essential oil

Instructions:

➢ Mix all ingredients until combined.
➢ Gently massage the scrub onto damp skin in circular motions.
➢ Rinse with warm water.

Benefits: Exfoliates dead skin cells, revealing smoother, healthier skin.

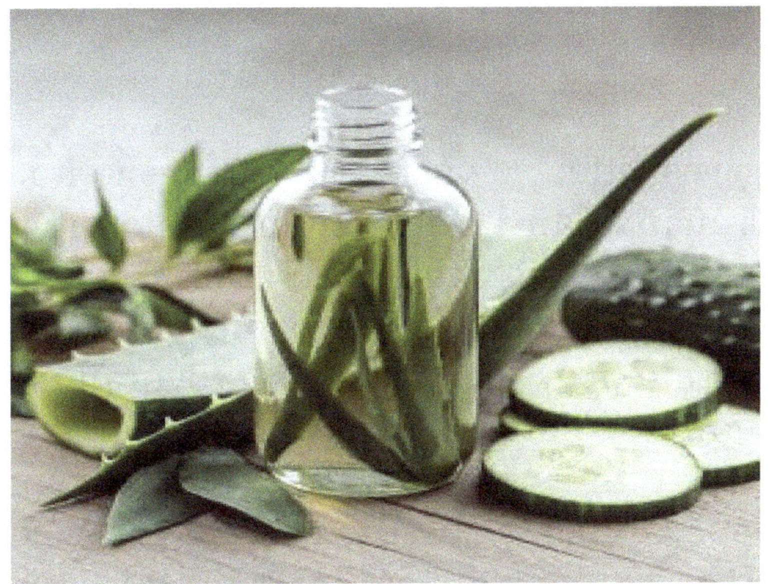

Refreshing Herbal Toner

Ingredients:

- ➢ 1 cup green tea (cooled)
- ➢ 1 tablespoon apple cider vinegar
- ➢ 1 teaspoon honey

Instructions:

- ➢ Combine all ingredients in a bottle and shake well.
- ➢ Use a cotton ball to apply the toner to your face after cleansing.

Benefits: This toner helps balance skin pH and refreshes the complexion.

By incorporating these DIY masks and tonics into your routine, you can customize your skincare while harnessing the power of herbs.

Conclusion

Herbs offer a vast array of benefits for skin and hair health. From promoting hair growth to treating specific skin conditions, integrating herbal remedies into your routine can enhance your overall well-being. Whether you choose to create herbal infusions, DIY masks, or topical applications, these natural remedies empower you to take control of your beauty regimen.

As you embark on your herbal journey, remember to listen to your body and skin. Each person's skin responds differently to various herbs, so it may take some experimentation to find what works best for you. Embrace the art of herbal healing and nurture your skin and hair naturally, allowing the gifts of nature to support your journey toward health and beauty

.

Chapter 10
Creating a Personalized Herbal Medicine Cabinet

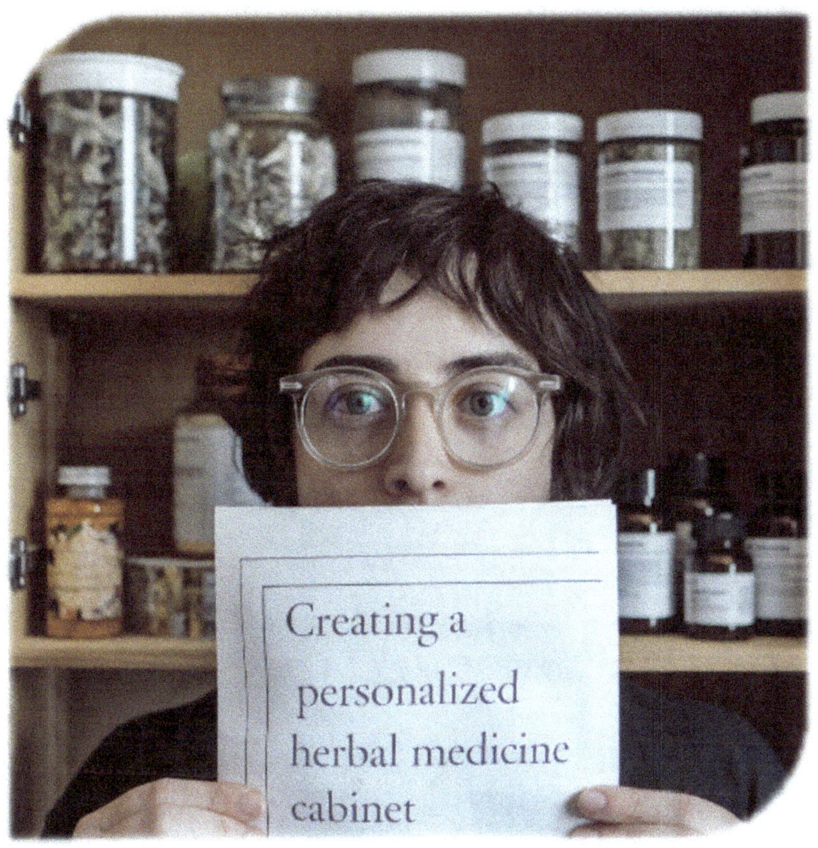

Creating a personalized herbal medicine cabinet is an empowering step toward taking charge of your health and well-being. A well-stocked herbal kit allows you to address common ailments naturally, tailor your remedies to your unique health concerns, and engage with your health on a deeper level. In this chapter, we'll explore essential herbs, organization techniques, and how to make informed decisions about your herbal practices.

To begin your herbal journey, it's important to have a foundational collection of herbs that can help address common ailments. Here are the must-have herbs for your herbal medicine cabinet:

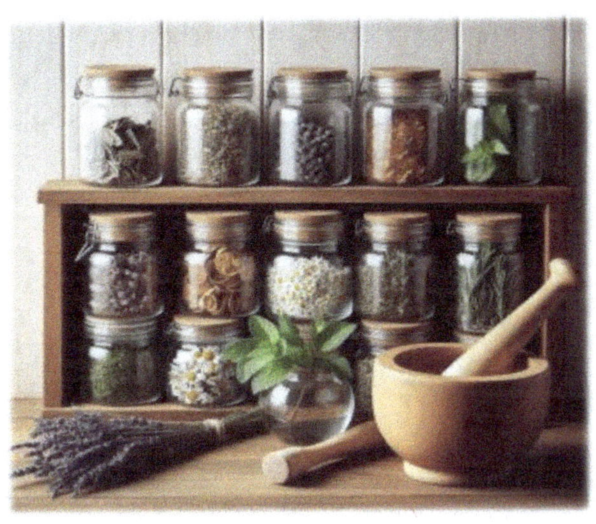

1. Echinacea

Uses: Known for its immune-boosting properties, echinacea is ideal for colds, flu, and respiratory infections.

How to Use: Take as a tincture, tea, or in capsules. It's best used at the onset of symptoms for maximum effectiveness.

2. Ginger

Uses: Ginger is excellent for digestive issues, nausea, and inflammation.

How to Use: Use fresh ginger in teas, smoothies, or meals. Dried ginger powder can be added to capsules or brewed as tea.

3. Turmeric

Uses: Renowned for its anti-inflammatory properties, turmeric supports joint health and can aid in digestion.

How to Use: Incorporate into cooking, take as a supplement, or make turmeric tea with black pepper to enhance absorption.

4. Chamomile

Uses: Chamomile is calming and can help with sleep, anxiety, and digestive upset.

How to Use: Brew chamomile tea or use chamomile essential oil in a diffuser for relaxation.

5. Peppermint

Uses: Peppermint is beneficial for digestive discomfort and headaches.

How to Use: Brew peppermint tea or use peppermint essential oil for topical relief or aromatherapy.

6. Lavender

Uses: Lavender is known for its soothing properties and can help with stress, anxiety, and sleep disturbances.

How to Use: Use lavender essential oil in a diffuser, apply diluted oil to the skin, or brew lavender tea.

7. Garlic

Uses: Garlic has antimicrobial properties and is beneficial for cardiovascular health and immune support.

How to Use: Incorporate fresh garlic into cooking or take garlic supplements.

By starting with these core herbs, you'll be well-equipped to handle a variety of common health issues.

Adapting to Your Unique Needs

Every individual has different health concerns and needs. Tailoring your herbal medicine cabinet to reflect your unique health profile is crucial. Consider the following steps:

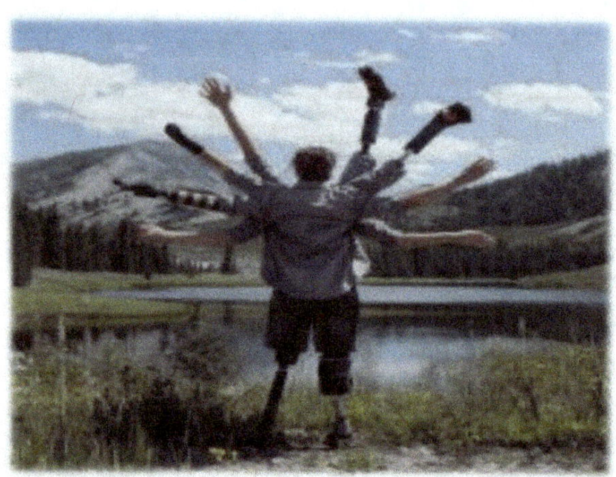

1. Assess Your Health Goals

➢ Identify your specific health concerns, such as digestive issues, immune support, or stress management.
➢ Consider any chronic conditions you may have, as some herbs can complement conventional treatments.

2. Research Herbs for Your Needs

➢ Investigate herbs known to support your health goals. For example:
➢ For anxiety: Look into ashwagandha or lemon balm.
➢ For digestive support: Consider fennel or licorice root.

3.Consult Reliable Resources

➤ Seek advice from trusted books, online resources, or experienced herbalists to learn more about the herbs that suit your needs.

4. Experiment Gradually

➤ Introduce new herbs one at a time to observe how your body responds. This approach helps you understand which herbs work best for you and allows you to track their effects.

Adapting your herbal kit to your specific needs ensures that you have the most relevant remedies at your fingertips.

When to Grow vs. When to Buy

Understanding when to grow your own herbs and when to purchase them is essential for building your herbal medicine cabinet. Here are some considerations:

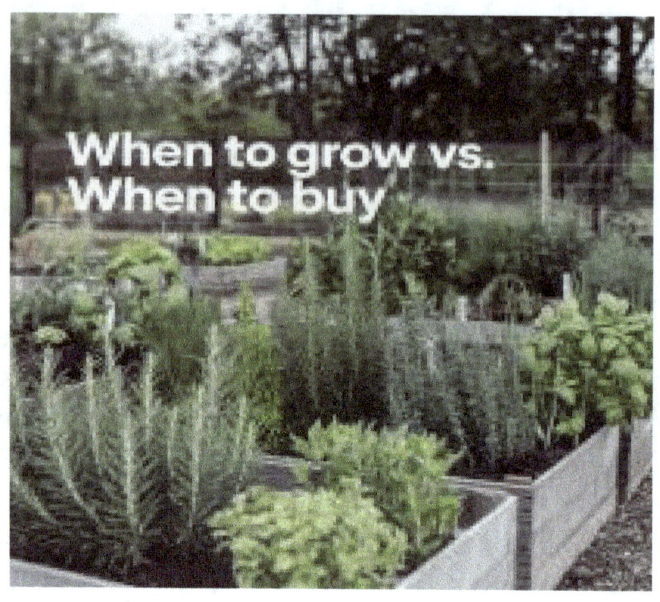

- **Growing Your Own Herbs**

  - **Benefits**: Growing your own herbs allows you to ensure quality, control growing conditions, and save money.
  - **Ideal Herbs**: Start with easy-to-grow herbs such as basil, mint, and rosemary, which can thrive in pots on a balcony or windowsill.

- **When to Buy Herbs**

  - **Considerations**:

  - **Space and Time**: If you lack outdoor space or time to tend to a garden, purchasing dried herbs or herbal products is a practical solution.

➢ **Specialized Herbs**: Some herbs may not be easily grown in your region or require specific growing conditions (like echinacea or calendula).

➢ **Quality Matters**: When purchasing, choose organic or sustainably sourced products to ensure potency and purity.

By evaluating your circumstances, you can make informed decisions about growing versus buying herbs for your medicine cabinet.

Organizing and Storing Your Herbal Remedies

An organized herbal medicine cabinet allows for easy access and ensures your herbs remain effective. Here are some best practices for organization and storage:

● Create a Dedicated Space

➢ Designate a specific area for your herbal remedies, whether it's a shelf, cabinet, or drawer. Ensure this space is cool, dark, and dry to maintain herb potency.

● Label Everything

➢ Clearly label jars, containers, or bags with the herb name, date of purchase, and any other relevant information (like dosage instructions). This will help you easily identify and track your herbs.

● Use Airtight Containers

➢ Store herbs in airtight containers to protect them from moisture, light, and air. Glass jars, amber bottles, or vacuum-sealed bags work well.

● Keep a Log

➢ Maintain a log or journal of your herbal remedies, noting when you purchased or harvested each herb, how you use it, and any observed effects.

By following these organizational strategies, you'll ensure that your herbal medicine cabinet remains a valuable resource for your health needs.

Tracking Your Herbal Use

Keeping a record of your herbal use is crucial for understanding what works for you. Here's how to create an effective tracking system:

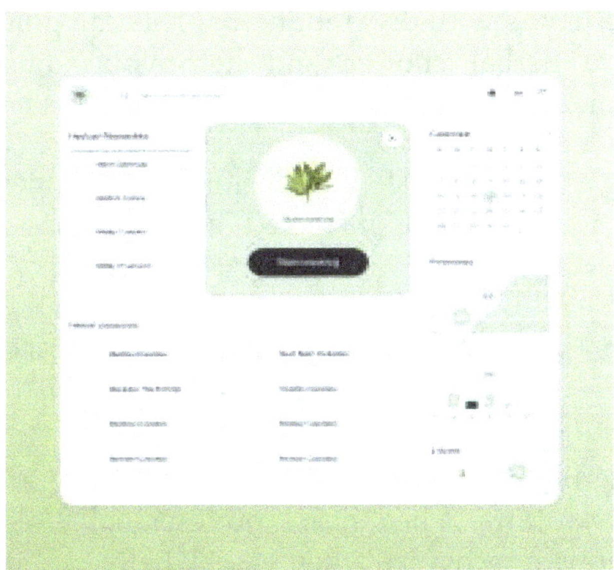

● Start a Herbal Journal

Dedicate a notebook or digital document to track your herbal remedies. Include sections for:

➢ Herb names
➢ Dosages taken
➢ Symptoms or conditions treated
➢ Observations or effects noticed

● Be Consistent

➢ Record your herbal use regularly, especially when trying new herbs or adjusting dosages. Consistency will help you identify patterns and assess the effectiveness of your remedies.

- ## Reflect on Your Experience

> ➤ Periodically review your journal to reflect on your experiences with different herbs. This can guide your future herbal choices and help you adjust your regimen as needed.

Tracking your herbal use fosters mindfulness and enables you to make informed decisions about your health.

Knowing When to Seek Professional Help

While herbal remedies can be powerful, there are times when consulting a healthcare professional is essential. Here's how to recognize when to seek help:

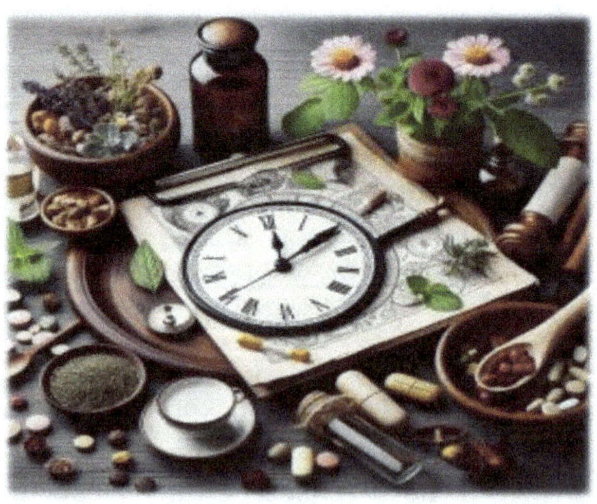

- ## Persistent Symptoms

> If you experience ongoing or worsening symptoms despite using herbal remedies, it's crucial to consult a doctor or herbalist.

• Severe Reactions

> If you experience severe allergic reactions, unusual side effects, or any concerning symptoms after taking an herb, seek immediate medical attention.

• Conflicting Health Issues

> If you have chronic health conditions or are taking prescription medications, consult a healthcare professional before starting herbal remedies. Some herbs can interact with medications.

• Lack of Improvement

> If you do not notice any improvement after a reasonable time frame (usually several weeks) of using a specific herb, consider seeking guidance.

Understanding when to seek professional help ensures you receive appropriate care while still benefiting from herbal remedies.

Conclusion

Creating a personalized herbal medicine cabinet is an enriching journey that empowers you to take control of your health and wellness. By selecting core herbs, adapting to your unique needs, and organizing your remedies effectively, you can build a valuable resource for addressing common ailments naturally. Tracking your herbal use and recognizing when to seek professional help will enhance your experience and ensure safety.

As you embark on this herbal journey, remember that patience and experimentation are key. Allow yourself the grace to explore and learn, discovering the herbs that resonate with your body and lifestyle. With dedication and curiosity, your herbal medicine cabinet can become a trusted companion in your quest for health and well-being.

www.ingramcontent.com/pod-product-compliance
Lightning Source LLC
Chambersburg PA
CBHW061343250726
48657CB00004B/1311